Community
Pro
Health Visitors
Handbook

EDITED BY JACKIE CARNELL AND ROGER KLINE

RADCLIFFE MEDICAL PRESS

Radcliffe Medical Press Ltd
18 Marcham Road, Abingdon, Oxon OX14 1AA

British Library Cataloguing in Publication Data

A catalogue record for this book is available from the British Library.

ISBN 1 85775 371 2

Typeset by Action Publishing Technology, Gloucester
Printed and bound by Biddles Ltd, Guildford and King's Lynn

Contents

Preface

The changes taking place in community health and primary care services are little short of a revolution for community nurses.

Major changes in the ways in which service priorities are set, how the quality and effectiveness of services are developed, measured and monitored, and how staff are treated are underway. More changes will follow as primary care trusts gradually replace primary care groups and as the long-term process of moving the entire health service to a more public health, primary care-focused service takes place.

Almost one thousand community nurses are on the boards of primary care groups. Thousands more are directly involved in discussions regarding new structures as members of local nursing forums, as local accredited representatives of trade unions and professional organisations, and as managers.

This is the best opportunity since the formation of the NHS for community nurses to influence the directions, priorities and culture of the service.

This book is written to encourage and inform that process. It is written by practical experts who have hands-on experience of the radical changes underway.

It is written for every nurse working in community health and primary care who wishes to understand the changes and who wants to influence them. It is a practical book for health professionals who deliver the service.

Jackie Carnell
Roger Kline
March 1999

List of contributors

Barrie Brown
Regional Officer (North & Eastern Area)
MSF

Jackie Carnell
Director
Community Practitioners' and Health Visitors' Association

Rosemary Cook
Freelance writer
Medical, nursing and management issues

Denise Hagel
Director of Quality Improvement
Essex Rivers Healthcare

Annette Keen
Nursing Development Specialist
Practices made Perfect Ltd

Roger Kline
Head of Labour Relations
Community Practitioners' and Health Visitors' Association

Patricia Oakley
Director
Practices made Perfect Ltd

Thelma Sackman
Consultant
Primary care and nursing

1

Introduction

Rosemary Cook

The purpose of this chapter is to bring together and examine the many documents and papers relating to the latest changes to the health service. It will also identify the significance of the changes they introduce, and their combined impact on the service and those who work in it. A more detailed discussion of what these changes mean for health visitors and community practitioners is contained in subsequent chapters.

Background – 'The third way'

Prior to the General Election of 1997, the manifesto of the Labour Party outlined plans to reform some aspects of the National Health Service. Two of the most significant changes promised were the end of GP fundholding and the abolition of the 'internal market' in healthcare.

Seven months after the election of the Labour Party to Government, the Secretary of State for Health published a White Paper, *The New NHS: modern, dependable*, which heralded the start of the process of reform. It fulfilled the pre-election promises to end GP fundholding and the internal market. But it did not simply return the health service to the status quo which had existed before the market was introduced in the reforms of the early 1990s.

Instead, it claimed to introduce a 'third way' of running the NHS, between the extremes of the 'command and control' systems of the 1970s and the 'divisive internal market system' of the 1990s. It is the nuts and bolts of the 'third way' which make these changes the most significant to affect the health service, and the nurses who work within it, for many years.

Introducing the changes

The White Paper was followed by a range of other documents which expanded on the process and timetable for the implementation of the planned changes, and filled in operational details. They also linked the changes to other major health themes, such as public health and performance measurement in the NHS.

The scope and significance of the changes introduced by these documents must not be under-estimated. The 'new NHS' involves radical changes in the structure, funding and quality measurement of the entire service, and will significantly and permanently alter professional relationships and roles. It is essential that community practitioners have a clear understanding of the content and significance of these documents if they are to understand the impact that the changes will make on their daily professional lives. The most important documents were:

- a Green Paper (for consultation) on public health, *Our Healthier Nation*, in February 1998

- a number of health service circulars (HSCs) describing the implementation of the changes

- a consultation paper on proposed new quality indicators for the health service, *A Framework for Assessing Performance*

- a consultation paper on quality aspects of the 'new NHS', *A First Class Service*

- a new human resources strategy for the NHS called *Working Together*.

The status and content of these documents is shown in Table 1.1. The changes to the health service introduced by these documents fall into four categories:

- changes to structure
- changes to quality mechanisms
- changes to funding
- changes to professional roles and relationships.

Changes to structure: the system

The New NHS: modern, dependable replaces the internal market by a system 'based on partnership and driven by performance'. This change from a competitive internal market to a system of collaborative planning and commissioning involves:

- the production of collaborative 'Health Improvement Programmes' (HImPs) for all districts (*see* Box 1.1)
- long-term service agreements between NHS trusts and commissioners, organised around care groups (e.g. children) or disease areas (e.g. heart disease) in place of annual contracts
- a 'duty of partnership' on all NHS trusts
- a requirement on all health authorities to work with local authorities' social care services and 'all local interests', including hospital clinicians, in drawing up HImPs.

In line with these changes, the terms 'purchasing' and 'purchasers' have been replaced by 'commissioning' and 'commissioners'.

Changes to structure: the commissioners

In the internal market, the 'purchasers' of healthcare were either GP fundholders or health authorities (for populations not registered with a fundholding practice). With 100 health authorities in

Table 1.1 Status and content of major documents

Document	Status (as at 1.9.98)	CONTENT					
		Structure of new NHS	Quality mechanisms	Funding	Public health targets	Nurses in PCG commissioning	Timetable for implementation
The New NHS: modern, dependable	White Paper	✓	✓	✓		✓	
Our Healthier Nation	Green Paper (for consultation)		✓	✓	✓		
A National Framework for Assessing Performance	Consultation document		✓				
HSC 1998/021	Health service circular	✓					✓
HSC 1998/065	Health service circular	✓		✓		✓	✓
HSC 1998/121	Health service circular	✓		✓		✓	✓
HSC 1998/139	Health service circular	✓		✓		✓	✓
A First Class Service: quality in the new NHS	Consultation document		✓				✓
HSC 1998/162	Health service circular	✓				✓	
HSC 1998/to be numbered	Draft health service circular			✓		✓	

Box 1.1: The Health Improvement Programme

The HImP:
- is a local strategy for improving health and healthcare
- is developed by health authority in consultation with local trusts, primary care groups, other professionals such as dentists and pharmacists, the public and other partner organisations
- covers a three-year period, and part is updated each year
- covers the main health needs and healthcare requirements of local people, and the investment required in local health services to meet these needs
- includes targets from *Our Healthier Nation* and the National Framework for Assessing Performance
- is binding on the primary care groups and trusts in the area

---

England, and around 3500 fundholders, there were 3600 different purchasers in the system. The abolition of fundholding and the setting up of larger groups of commissioning practices – 'primary care groups' (PCGs) (*see* Box 1.2) – means:

- the number of commissioning bodies (PCGs) will eventually be around 500

- all GPs are involved in PCGs (unlike fundholding, participation will not be voluntary)

- PCGs are accountable to health authorities

- health authorities will gradually cease to be commissioners for most services, and will combine into fewer, larger authorities.

PCGs start at one of two levels, with progression to more independent levels planned for the future (*see* Box 1.3). Each PCG has a governing board with both professional and lay membership (*see* Box 1.4). In addition to these board members, PCGs can 'co-opt' members with relevant expertise. They are also required to consult with relevant professionals about particular services: for example, by involving midwives in the planning of maternity services. In some areas, local nursing groups have been set up to act as professional support to the nurse members of the PCG board.

Box 1.2: Characteristics of primary care groups

PCGs:
- include all GP practices within the boundaries of the group, as agreed with the local health authority and relevant regional office
- are subcommittees of the health authority, so the PCG chair is accountable to the chief executive of the health authority
- take responsibility for commissioning health services for their local community
- enter into long-term (3–5 year) 'service agreements' with NHS trusts for health services
- are responsible for promoting the health of local people, in partnership with other agencies; developing primary care services; and integrating primary and community health services more closely with social services, in planning and delivery

---

Box 1.3: The four 'levels' of primary care groups

Level 1   PCG acts in an advisory capacity to the health authority in commissioning care for its population

Level 2   PCG takes devolved responsibility for managing the budget for healthcare in its area

Level 3*   PCG is a free-standing body, accountable to the health authority for commissioning care

Level 4*   PCG is a free-standing body, accountable to the health authority for commissioning care, and with responsibility for providing community services for its population

*Levels 3 and 4 are a new kind of NHS trust – primary care trusts – which need new legislation to set up (*see* Chapter 6)

The functions of the PCG are:

- to contribute to the health authority's HImP

- to promote the health of the local population

- to commission health services for their local population from

Box 1.4: Primary care group boards

Designation	Number of repesentatives	Method of selection
GPs	4–7	Election
Community nurses*	1–2	Election or selection
Social services officer	1	Nomination by local authority
Lay member	1	Nomination by health authority
Health authority non-executive member	1	Nominated by HA
PCG chief officer (ex-officio (non-voting) member)	1	Appointed by the Board

*Community nurses were offered the chance to decide locally whether there should be one or two nurse members of the PCG board, and whether they should be selected through a ballot of volunteers, through a process of application and selection involving health authorities, or by a combination of these methods

NHS trusts, within the framework of the HImP

- to monitor performance against the service agreements

- to develop primary care by joint working across practices, sharing skills, professional development, audit and peer review, quality assurance and developing 'clinical governance' (see below)

- to influence the deployment of resources for general practice locally

- to better integrate primary and community health services, and work closely with social services on planning and delivery of care.

PCGs are accountable to their local health authority, through the lines of accountability shown in Figure 1.1.

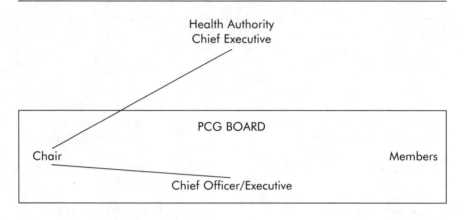

———— = accountability

Figure 1.1 PCG's accountability.

Significance of changes to structure

The most significant consequences of these changes to the health service are:

- PCGs bring GPs, who have always been (and remain) independent contractors rather than employees of the health service, into accountable, health service organisations for the first time
- general practices are required to work collaboratively, sharing information and undertaking joint planning and development, for the first time
- social services representatives and service user representatives will be formally involved with GPs and others in the planning and commissioning of local healthcare services
- community nurses will be formally involved in these processes for the first time.

Changes to quality mechanisms

In the market-led NHS, chief executives of NHS trusts had a statutory responsibility only for financial control. *The New NHS* placed a new statutory responsibility for the quality of care on trust chief executives. This statutory duty is backed by a new framework of organisations and processes to set and monitor quality standards (*see* Figure 1.2). The aims of this framework are:

- 'to match consistency in quality across the NHS with sensitivity to the needs of the individual patient and local community'
- to set clear national standards, with responsibility for delivery being taken locally, and backed by consistent monitoring arrangements.

Standards will be set through National Service Frameworks and through the new National Institute for Clinical Excellence (*see* Box 1.5). They will be delivered through a new system of 'clinical governance'. Standards will be monitored through three new mechanisms:

- the Commission for Health Improvement (CHI; *see* Box 1.6)
- a National Framework for Assessing Performance
- an annual National Survey of Patient and User Experience of the NHS.

National Service Frameworks –

- will set national service standards and define service models for a specific service or care group (coronary heart disease and mental health will be the first areas)
- will put in place programmes to support implementation
- will establish performance measures for the service
- will set out where care is best provided and the standard of care that patients should be offered

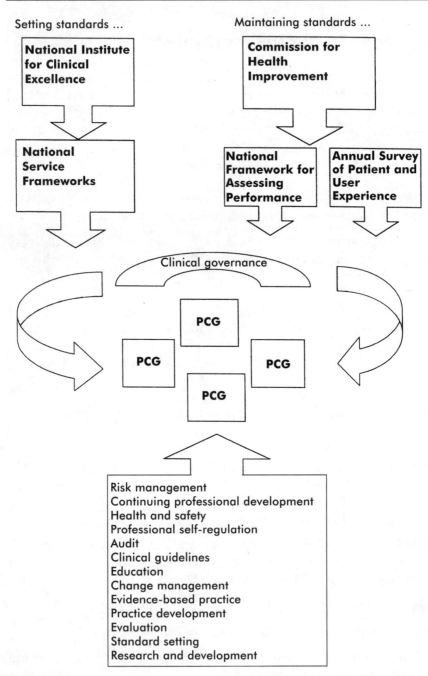

Figure 1.2 The quality framework in *The New NHS*.

Box 1.5: The National Institute for Clinical Excellence (NICE)

NICE:
- is a special health authority set up in 1999
- promotes clinical and cost-effectiveness through guidance and audit, and advises on best practice
- produces and disseminates clinical guidelines and associated clinical audit methodologies
- commissions and oversees functions previously undertaken by the National Centre for Clinical Audit, the National Guidelines Programme and the Effectiveness Bulletins
- gives patients and the wider public access to its information on health and best treatment through the Internet and digital television

Box 1.6: The Commission for Health Improvement

The CHI:
- is a new, independent, statutory body, to be set up in 1999/2000 through new legislation
- supports and oversees NHS activity, to assure and improve quality
- independently scrutinises local clinical governance arrangements through a rolling programme of reviews of service providers, visiting every trust over 3–4 years
- will visit a trust sooner if problems are identified by a regional office
- concentrates on clinical issues, but can be involved in management issues where these lie behind clinical problems
- can be asked to look at a trust's services by a health authority, regional office or service provider
- has powers to look at PCGs and health authorities if their actions are impacting on the issues being examined

- will bring together the best evidence of clinical and cost-effectiveness with the views of service users to determine the best ways of providing particular services.

Clinical governance is a framework through which NHS organisations are accountable for continuously improving the quality of their services'. It has clinical audit and evidence-based practice as a 'key component but also includes all professional activities aimed at maintaining and improving care. Examples are activities which:

- identify and build on good practice (e.g. research, bench-marking, standard setting)

- assess and minimise the risk of untoward events (risk manage-ment, health and safety activity)

- investigate problems as they arise and ensure lessons are learnt (e.g. complaints handling)

- support health professionals in delivering quality care (e.g. continuing professional development, staff support activities).

Every PCG has a nominated doctor or nurse taking lead responsi-bility for clinical governance, and the production of an annual accountability report.

The National Framework for Assessing Performance focuses on six main areas of the health service (*see* Box 1.7). It sets indicators in each area, and data are gathered at health authority level on each indicator. The intention is that results can be used to look at perfor-mance of the NHS in different 'dimensions': by population group (e.g. children or the elderly); by disease area; by health authority, primary care group or trust; or by service (e.g. orthopaedics or mental health). A small set of 'high level indicators', which is not intended to be comprehensive and uses only currently available data, is used to compare performance in different health authority

---

Box 1.7: The National Framework for Assessing Performance key areas

The key areas are:
- health improvement
- fair access to services
- effective delivery of appropriate healthcare
- efficiency
- patient and carer experience
- health outcomes of NHS care

areas. Some of these indicators are particularly relevant to primary care, including:

- fair access – access to family planning services, early detection of breast and cervical cancer, district nurse contacts

- effective delivery of appropriate healthcare – disease prevention (through immunisation), early detection of breast and cervical cancer, surgical intervention for glue ear, hospital admissions for acute conditions (severe ENT infection, kidney/urinary tract infection, heart failure) and chronic conditions (asthma, diabetes, epilepsy), volume of benzodiazepine prescribing

- health outcomes – conceptions in under-16s, tooth decay in under-5-year-olds, avoidable diseases (pertussis, measles, tuberculosis), fractures of proximal femur, infant deaths.

The National Survey of Patient and User Experience has been developed by a specialist survey provider and aims to cover the areas which patients identify as important in the service they receive. The survey is carried out annually and samples views from each health district. The results are published in annual reports and focus on local performance, compared both over time and with other areas. All local NHS organisations have to show their NHS Executive Regional Office how they have addressed the issues raised by the patient survey. The 1998 survey included specific questions on people's experiences of primary and community care.

Significance of changes to quality mechanisms

The most significant consequences of these changes are:

- quality issues in trusts will be given the same weight as financial issues because of the new statutory duty for quality

- the quality of care provided by GPs and their primary health-care teams will come under the scrutiny of the PCG

- individual practices and practitioners will be required to share more information, and work together more closely than ever before, on quality improvement programmes such as audit and peer review

- practices or teams which are 'outliers' in terms of quality within the PCG can expect to be identified and scrutinised by the group's nominated clinical governance lead.

Changes to funding

Prior to the changes introduced by *The New NHS*, the money allocated to health authorities was divided into three separate budgets:

- HCHS (used to purchase hospital and community health services)

- GMS (General Medical Services) cash-limited, to fund individual GP practice infrastructure: for example, staffing, premises and computer developments

- GMS non-cash-limited, used to fund prescribing.

GPs in the standard fundholding scheme received their share of each of these budgets to spend on their registered patient population.

In the 'new NHS', health authorities receive a single, cash-limited, unified budget, covering HCHS, GMS cash-limited and prescribing. From this allocation, health authorities agree a unified budget for each primary care group, with the aim of achieving a 'fair shares' allocation based on a national formula (*see* Figure 1.3). Health authorities can, after discussion with local PCGs, deduct some funding prior to this allocation to PCGs, to cover specialist services, health authority functions and agreed collaborative commissioning undertaken at health authority level

One proviso on the 'unified' budget for PCGs is the setting of an expenditure 'floor' for cash-limited GMS at health authority level designed to protect the current level of investment in practice

Before the new NHS ...

HCHS	GMS (cash-limited for practice staff computers and premises)	GMS (non cash-limited for prescribing)

After the new NHS ...

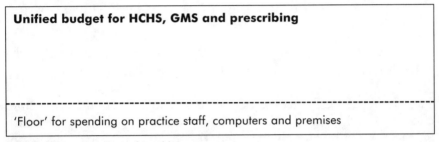

Figure 1.3   Funding of healthcare.

infrastructure. This also ensures that there is a guarantee of sufficient funding for the reimbursement of current practice staff posts, as well as computer maintenance.

Over time, it is expected that PCG boards will further allocate their funds by giving 'indicative', or theoretical, budgets to individual practices in the group. Initially, each practice will have its own prescribing budget.

PCGs and their money

There are some ground rules for the way in which a PCG uses its budget. These include the requirements for each PCG to:

• manage within its budget: in addition, however, the guidance makes it clear that 'the freedom to refer and prescribe remains unchanged. Patients will continue to be guaranteed the drugs, investigations and treatments they need'. PCGs will have to manage the conflict of interest which may arise from a cash-limited budget and an unlimited guarantee

• ensure fairness between practices and patients (*see* primary care investment plans, below)

- work with other PCGs and the health authority to establish risk management strategies: this can include each PCG putting some money into a contingency reserve fund

- guarantee at least the existing level of investment in primary care (see below): there is a requirement to give one year's notice to practices of any change to existing commitments

- set up an incentive framework for practices within the PCG to promote better use of resources or improved clinical performance

- operate within the same statutory financial framework as the health authority, as a subcommittee of the health authority.

The chairs of PCGs are accountable to the health authority chief executive, who has a statutory duty under the National Health Service Act 1977 to ensure that the health authority does not exceed its cash limit. As the accountable officer, the chair will also be responsible for ensuring that the PCGs have robust financial management in place.

Primary care investment plans

Each PCG has to produce a costed primary care investment plan (PCIP) which covers:

- plans for GMS infrastructure developments – that is, investments in practice staff, computers and premises

- broader primary care developments, such as proposals for in-house services and the development of community nursing.

PCIPs are subject to health authority approval, but individual practices' proposals for new investment in practice staff, premises and computers are now submitted to the PCG board, for consideration in the PCIP, rather than direct to the health authority. The PCIP has particular significance for all community nurses, since this will be the instrument for bringing about changes in staffing, ways of working and future developments in both practice nursing and community nursing within the PCG.

Significance of changes to funding

The most significant consequences of these changes to funding are:

- unified budgets give PCGs the opportunity to move money traditionally used for hospital and community health services into other areas of health commissioning

- the cash limit on the whole budget, and the requirement to keep within that budget, means that PCG boards will have to take responsibility for rationing their limited cash, while trying to fulfil the commitment to prescribe and refer according to need

- the PCIP, drawn up by the PCG board, will decide on the level and extent of future investment in practice staff, including nurses, and the development of community nursing services.

Changes to professional roles and relationships

Before the latest changes brought about by *The New NHS*, trust-employed community nurses and practice nurses had two potentially challenging roles to reconcile. Both were part of a primary healthcare team, serving one or more general practice's registered patients. But in addition, community nurses and health visitors were part of a package of 'community nursing services' purchased by the health authority or by fundholding GPs. Their work was defined by the contract and measured by the agreed contract currency – often numbers of contacts with clients. Similarly, practice nurses combined their role as part of the primary healthcare team with being direct employees of one member of the team, the GP (*see* Figure 1.4). At worst, the practice nurse could choose to relate only to the GP, while the other community nurses focused only on their trust and the primary healthcare team would exist in name only.

In some places, the potential divisions caused by these differences are addressed by creating an 'integrated', self-managed primary healthcare team. A team leader or co-ordinator, appointed from within the team, takes managerial responsibility for the work, organisation and development of the team (*see* Figure 1.5).

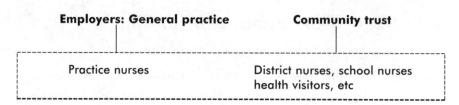

Figure 1.4 Community nursing before *The New NHS*.

Bringing together individual GP practices into primary care groups, with a governing body which includes community nurses, has had two major effects, to be managed together with the continuing differences between community and practice nurses outlined above.

PCGs:

- make all community and practice nurses, and health visitors, part of a new organisation, the PCG, but without changing their current employers

- give nurses and health visitors in 'front line' clinical posts the opportunity to become involved in commissioning and developing healthcare and health services for a community.

Nurses in PCGs

One of the roles of the PCG is 'to develop primary care by joint working across practices, sharing skills, audit and peer review...'. In order to achieve this, all community nurses and health visitors will have to work as part of the larger organisation, not just as part of one or more primary healthcare teams (*see* Figure 1.6). This

Employers: General practice   **Community trust**

> Team leader/Co-ordinator
>
> Practice nurses   District nurses   Health visitors
>
> Other nurses working with practice's patients

Figure 1.5 Integrated nursing teams.

could be regarded as one big 'integrated team'. PCGs have a huge and challenging list of tasks to accomplish, and cannot afford to allow any staff to distance themselves from the concerted effort to achieve them. Developing a 'corporate', pan-PCG culture and practice will be high on the list of things to do for the new PCGs.

Health visitors and community nurses have many of the vital skills necessary to the work of the PCG, including:

- community profiling
- health needs assessment
- client advocacy
- involving service users and other stakeholders
- assessing quality of services
- assessing user satisfaction with services
- piloting innovative practice
- managing chronic conditions
- developing services.

The PCG board will be looking to the nurses working within it to use these skills, particularly as it has practical, service priorities to address each year, for which it will be held accountable by the health authority.

Influence over the priorities, decisions and outcomes of the PCG's work is not only available to nurses who have a seat on the board of the PCG. Much of the work needed to inform the board's decision making about commissioning, service change and development will be undertaken by subgroups of appropriate professionals who report to the board.

Nurses on the PCG board

Nurses have up to two places on the board of each PCG, and others may be co-opted for their particular experience or expertise. They are chosen by a process of election, or appointment, or a combination of both methods. The constituency involved in the

---

Primary care group

Employers: All general practices   **Community trust**

All nursing teams from all practices
in primary care group

Figure 1.6   Nurses in primary care groups.

elections varied in different areas, but often included all nurses working in primary care, regardless of whether they were employed by a community or an acute trust. Mental health nurses, learning disability nurses and midwives were therefore able to take part in the elections, and in some places they have been elected to PCG boards.

The role of the board nurses is not to represent individual professional or clinical groups, but to bring the perspectives of nursing, midwifery or health visiting to the work of the board. As with other members of the board, they are required to act corporately rather than individually, to help the board achieve its tasks and responsibilities.

Nurses on PCG boards need to:

- find ways of consulting appropriate professional colleagues about issues and decisions, and reflecting that expertise back to the board

- develop skills in negotiation and facilitation, particularly important because of their minority on the board

- develop a strategic approach to their board responsibilities, accessing appropriate sources of information, objectively appraising the options and ensuring that they understand the 'big picture' as well as the individual pieces.

Significance of changes to community nursing

The most significant aspects of these changes are:

- nurses in individual primary healthcare teams or practices are now part of a larger organisation

- community nurses will have to work across the PCG to assess and develop services, and participate in quality assessment and improvement

- all community nurses can contribute to service change and development through work on subgroups of the PCG

- some 'front line' nurses will be directly involved in commissioning of health services for the first time

- nurses on PCG boards will be involved in 'rationing' decisions about the use of limited funding for health services.

Summary

- *The New NHS* introduces significant changes to every aspect of the health service.

- Community nurses are in the forefront of the changes, with decisions about commissioning and developing both primary and secondary health services made much closer to them and the public they work with.

- Community nurses have new opportunities to use their existing skills, and develop new skills, in the work of the PCGs.

2

Human resources in primary care

Barrie Brown and Roger Kline

'The Government has lost faith in the people. It is time to elect a new people.'

Bertolt Brecht

In recent years, it has felt to many staff that some politicians and trusts felt that if it wasn't for troublesome staff, they could run a really efficient health service. In the words of Labour's first Secretary of State for Health for 18 years, 'staff were often seen as part of the problem, not part of the solution'.

The publication of *The New NHS: modern, dependable* and especially *Working Together*, the Human Resources strategy for the NHS in England, signalled a change of direction. Partly driven by conviction, but also by necessity as staff shortages loomed, this approach provides the framework for the human resources challenge facing community nurses in primary care.

The human resources framework

This chapter sets out to summarise:

- the key statutory obligations NHS organisations have on quality which in turn enshrine existing obligations flowing from the duty of care and the public interest

- the statutory and common law duties faced by NHS organisations and employees in respect of employment rights

- the challenge for employers and primary care groups (PCGs) arising from the Human Resources (HR) framework for the NHS in England – including a Health Improvement Programme (HImP) for staff.

These requirements will in turn inform the central role of the HR strategy in England, *Working Together*, which is to:

- 'ensure that we have a quality workforce, in the right numbers with the right skills and diversity, organised in the right way, to deliver the Government's service objectives for health and social care'

- 'be able to demonstrate we are improving the quality of working life for staff'

- 'address the management capacity and capability required to deliver this agenda'.

The rest of this chapter takes the clinical care and quality, employment contract and quality of working life themes, and then considers the implications for both management and employees working within primary care. We do so in the light of the development of PCGs and primary care trusts (PCTs), bearing in mind a crucial objective of the HR strategy:

Each primary care group/primary care trust to demonstrate preparedness and commitment to sign up to the HR framework and meet the minimum standards on HR as set out in central guidance.

One look at the HR strategy (*see* Box 2.1) and the legal framework that underpins it makes clear how great a challenge that is.

> **Box 2.1:** Elements of the HR framework
>
> - Duty of clinical care
> - Employment rights and responsibilities
> - HR strategy including quality of working life
> - Role of trade unions and professional organisations

The duty of clinical care and quality

The only statutory duties placed upon NHS trusts until recently were financial – particularly the duty to break even. The Health Act sets out a parallel statutory obligation to provide quality care for patients and clients. This proposal anticipated the child heart surgery tragedy in United Bristol Hospitals Trust but its importance was already laid out in *A First Class Service*, which defines clinical governance and which Chapter 4 of this handbook discusses in some detail.

The Department of Health (DoH) now requires NHS organisations to put in place local working practices and audit processes which, linked to the National Institute of Clinical Excellence and the Commission for Health Improvement, will require them to have a named person to lead on quality with the buck stopping with the chief executive. These persons will need to put in place guidelines and protocols to ensure that:

- practice is increasingly evidence supported
- poor performance can be identified and tackled
- new procedures and new equipment meet the duty of quality
- all those working in the NHS are properly trained, updated, competent, safely and effectively managed and that these requirements are regularly audited
- openness and transparency in clinical practice become the norm with the right to whistleblow enshrined in statute.

The Health Act is complemented by the Public Interest Disclosure Act which provides statutory protection for whistleblowers under defined circumstances.

The statutory quality requirement on NHS organisations in turn complements the duties set out in the UKCC Code of Professional Conduct for the individual registered practitioner who must:

report to an appropriate person or authority, having regard to the physical, psychological and social effects on patients and clients, any circumstances in the environment of care which could jeopardise standards of practice

and

report to an appropriate person or authority any circumstances in which safe and appropriate care for patients and clients cannot be provided

and

acknowledge any limitations in your knowledge and competence and decline any duties or responsibilities unless able to perform them in a safe and skilled manner.

The Code is a summary of the duty of care owed. Registered nurses, midwives and health visitors cannot be required to, or offer to, breach that Code by act or omission, even where their immediate line manager, peer pressure or ignorance insists on this.

Most contracts of employment make it a serious disciplinary offence to breach the Code. Even where this is not so, whenever there is a management instruction requiring a breach of the Code this must be challenged as being a potential breach of the contract of employment.

Implications for management

The statutory duty places obligations on both management and staff. Management will need to:

- put in place the various guidelines and protocols – preceded by appropriate consultation

- be sure they are clear what the new statutory duty means and what the guidance on clinical governance requires of them

- be clear about their own professional accountability and that of staff they manage or commission services from and its implications for individual practice.

In doing so, they will need to ensure that in considering work-loads, skill mix, new procedures, protocols and guidance, training and continuing professional development (CPD), they observe the statutory and common law duties placed upon employers as a template against which such developments are monitored and evaluated.

Management at all levels must be given training so they are aware of their legal obligations and are able to implement the new arrangements. Each NHS organisation – NHS trusts, health authorities, PCGs, PCTs and GP practices – must set out in writing:

- what their arrangements are

- who they apply to

- who is responsible for what

- what training arrangements and CPD are to be put in place

- the consequences of not following these arrangements

- how they are to be monitored and evaluated

- the implications for the entire range for their management role – from workforce planning, through the management of change to disciplinary and capability procedures.

Individual managers at every level must ensure such arrangements are in place, that they are aware of them and understand them, and have the support and advice in place to enable them to safely adhere to them.

For nurse managers, of course, the obligations of the UKCC Code of Professional Conduct apply to them as much as to their staff.

These requirements apply to GPs in their management and employer roles.

Whilst the majority of GPs work in partnership, a significant number are single-handed. These GPs, for the most part, are to be found in socially deprived urban areas. Often they will lack the resources and management expertise which can be found in GP partnerships when addressing HR issues. Staff who work for single-handed GPs need to be aware of the problems this may present in ensuring their employment and related rights are guaranteed.

Management will need to ensure that the cost in management time and staff resources of meeting these requirements is acknowledged in the commissioning of services and the provision of budgets.

Implications for staff

Registered nurses have three obligations arising from their employment in the NHS:

- their duty of care to patients, clients, each other and themselves
- their professional accountability codified in the UKCC Code of Professional Conduct
- their duty to obey reasonable instructions.

Though these should never be in conflict, they sometimes are – as when staff are instructed to undertake, or agree to undertake:

- work they are not competent to do
- not to draw to the attention of appropriate persons breaches of their duty of care, the public interest or their Code of Professional Conduct
- excessive workloads with a consequent risk for the nature and quality of clinical services provided.

Common law, and the UKCC Code of Conduct, make it clear that it is no defence to negligence resulting from such acts or omissions to claim:

- you didn't know better, when you should have done

- you were instructed to, when that instruction was a breach of the duty of care or your Code of Professional Conduct

- pressure of work led you to your breach of your duty of care.

The framework of clinical governance directly impacts on these difficult issues. By making explicit the requirement to provide quality services, it obliges the employer and commissioner of services to take due account of them.

Staff – and their local representatives – are entitled to:

- be involved in developing the local clinical governance arrangements

- be formally consulted on proposals

- ensure they have the training, professional and management support needed to work safely and effectively

- insist that proposals to change skill mix use clinical governance as a template against which proposals are checked – especially where work may be delegated to persons not competent to undertake it

- insist that concerns about excessive workloads are taken seriously since staff with excessive workloads run the risk of working ineffectively and unsafely

- insist that their employer remove all gagging clauses in accordance with the Public Disclosure Act, ministerial guidance and spirit and the intention of the Health Act – and put in place clear procedures to whistleblow within their employment

- insist that arrangements for clinical support and advice are informed by consideration of quality and safe practice

- ensure that, in accordance with *Working Together*,

  'each local employer has in place training and development plans for the majority of health professional staff' and that these are fully funded by the employer. There should be no question of any member of staff being expected to meet the cost of course fees and attending courses.'

As well as such requirements applying to employers (e.g. NHS trusts and GP practices) they also form a central consideration in decision making at PCG boards.

Local representatives will need to ensure that a formal agreement setting out this framework is consulted on and agreed with them on behalf of staff. It will not be acceptable, whether in NHS trusts, PCGs or GP practices for employers and commissioners of services to refuse to discuss these matters formally with staff representatives.

Local representatives will need to ensure that the clinical governance framework is one that first looks at systemic issues – shortcomings in the organisation – rather than uses clinical governance to primarily tackle individual failings. Individual failings must be tackled, but experience within the NHS suggests that this must go hand in hand with a systemic approach, not be a cheap alternative to tackling deep-rooted organisational weaknesses.

Employment rights

A complex, and changing, framework of employment rights exists for employees in the NHS. As we went to press, further important legislative changes were being introduced such as:

• the Employment Rights Bill

• the Human Rights Act

• the Protection from Harassment Act

• the Working Time Directive and regulations

• EC directives on parental leave.

In addition, the Courts were improving the rights of part-time workers and the rights of workers being transferred between employers.

A framework of employment rights for NHS organisations will need several strands to meet the legal duties placed upon employers:

- fair and due process in *entry* to employment – including how the advertising, shortlisting, interviews and appointments procedures work. *Working Together* requires local employers to 'demonstrate progress towards a workforce that year on year becomes more representative of the community it serves at all levels of the organisation'

- fair and due process in *treatment* during employment – in respect of discrimination, harassment, bullying, stress, safe practice, CPD and training, and transfers. *Working Together* requires local employers to 'have policies and procedures in place to tackle harassment by staff and service users supported by monitoring and reporting arrangements to measure progress'

- fair and due process in *disciplinary and capability* procedures – including their being equality proofed in content and operation

- fair and due process regarding the *health and safety* of employees (as well as the public). This would need to take account of an extensive raft of legislation, now complemented by clear guidance from the NHS Executive on the importance of having in place clear policies and procedures, clear lines of accountability, training and risk management systems. This should dovetail with a wide range of rights for staff representatives to inspect premises, be consulted on health and safety issues, and be properly informed. The prosecution and subsequent resignation of the chief executive of one trust for failure to have a policy in place has certainly concentrated minds. In addition, *Working Together* has three specific health and safety goals requiring employers to

> 'have systems in place to record and monitor workplace accidents and violence against staff and have published strategies to achieve a reduction of such incidents'

> 'achieve year on year improvement in sickness absence rates'

> 'have in place Occupational Health Services and counselling available for all staff'

- fair and due process in respect of the *exit* of staff from jobs and employment whether through redundancy, dismissal or transfer
- fair and due process to determine the *pay, terms and conditions* of employees including a commitment to a national pay system and an equal pay proofed pay structure (*see* Box 2.2).

Box 2.2: Community nurses and pay

The formation of PCGs will make no difference at all to the pay arrangements of community nurses:

- most trust nurses are paid on Whitley scales – via the Nursing & Midwifery Staffs Negotiating Council Clinical Grading Structure
- a minority of trust nurses are paid on local trust job evaluation schemes
- the very small number of nurses employed by health authorities are employed on the NMNC Clinical Grading Structure scales or on Senior Management Pay or Administrative and Clerical staff pay scales
- practice nurses generally have their pay linked to the NMNC Clinical Grading Structure scales, though often without being on the right scale or increment or without London weighting

The formation of PCTs might make a difference, but this will not be clear until much nearer the formation of PCTs and may depend on progress towards a new pay system for all NHS staff

---

All aspects of these policies, of course, should be scrutinised to ensure equality of opportunity. All primary care employers, including GPs, can expect to provide the same workforce census statistical information as the rest of the NHS to enable progress to be monitored locally and nationally.

In addition the DoH is committed to a programme of Social Partnership to involve staff and their representatives, including trade unions, who are recognised as stakeholders in this whole process:

the new NHS calls for greater staff involvement and participation in service development and planning change.

These employment rights have been embraced by the new HR strategy not simply because they are entitlements but because of a recognition that at a time of:

• labour shortages in many professions

• rapid change in services and service delivery

• low morale amongst many staff

it becomes a 'business necessity' to put in place fair and equitable working arrangements and procedures as a key part of attracting and retaining skilled staff.

This is further examined below in the section on the quality of working life.

There are some differences between the implications of this framework for staff depending on their employment contract.

As Box 2.3 shows, there are three main types of contract of employment in primary care, excluding GPs who are not employees, agency and contractor staff. Whereas Whitley contracts cannot be amended in any significant way by the local employer, general practice contracts and some trust contracts can be, although, in fact, the majority of trust contracts 'mirror' Whitley in almost all respects.

Box 2.3: Different employment contracts in primary care	
NHS trust staff	two-thirds on Whitley contracts
Health authority staff	only on Whitley contracts
PCG staff	probably on health authority Whitley contracts
Practice staff and GP assistants	almost all on practice contracts
GPs and GP partners	self-employed except for salaried GPs

Implications for management

The HR strategy seeks to have a motivated, flexible workforce, capable of responding to and driving different priorities, and the means of delivering services. To do this at a time of limited financial and staffing resources means there will be pressure:

- to introduce *skill mix* where this can be done without reducing quality and safe practice

- to introduce *efficiency savings* at all levels

- to *restructure services* in a way that makes staff more flexible but guarantees no one should be compulsorily redundant and all staff get the opportunity to constantly update old skills and learn new ones

- to review *workforce planning and training priorities* in the light of changing health service priorities.

Those pressures will shape much of the work of PCGs and PCTs.

One has only to list the legal requirements which underpin the employment contract to recognise how far some employers are from what is expected. At the same time all NHS employers have to have due regard to their legal obligations as tested in the Employment Tribunals and Courts.

It is essential that management has in place clear, published policies and procedures to implement all these elements of the employment contract. These policies and procedures must make it clear:

- who is responsible for implementing each policy

- what the responsibilities of middle and junior management are

- that all management will be trained and have support and advice in their role

- that there are means of complaining about breaches of these policies, and all terms within the contract, including where necessary the application of the grievance procedure

- how they are monitored and evaluated, and by whom, including their equal opportunities implications.

In the light of the Social Partnership, it may be assumed that trade union recognition will be the norm and that such agreements:

- will not be restrictive in terms of the range of membership covered or issues which may be raised

- will provide for appropriate time off, cover, facilities and training for local representatives

- will recognise all trade unions with membership within that organisation.

In addition to formal negotiating and consultation arrangements within each employer, there should also be established a health authority forum to discuss and agree issues arising from the work of PCGs, including the HR issues.

These arrangements should apply to all staff working within the NHS and not just those employed by health authorities and trusts. These will include agency and bank staff, contract staff, temporary staff, staff with PFI schemes and especially staff within GP practices.

Implications for staff

The employment framework set out above should be summarised in the individual written contract of employment which every employee is entitled to receive within two months of starting work. A surprising number of NHS employees – particularly practice staff – do not receive their legal entitlement to the statement of their main terms of employment.

Every employee is entitled to a written statement of employment setting out the job title, exact salary, working hours, holiday entitlement and pay, as well as having access to documents setting out sick leave entitlements and arrangements, pension arrangements, notice period, grievance procedures and (where there are more than 20 employees) the disciplinary procedure. This is commonly regarded as the contract of employment.

If you do not have a written contract, this doesn't mean you don't have a contract of employment, but it does mean there may be confusion over what your rights and responsibilities are. So it is important to get one, if necessary by exercising your legal right to obtain one under the current employment rights legislation.

It is not necessary for each member of staff to have a complete set of all agreements, procedures and policies. Indeed that would probably not be practical. What is important is that every employee knows that they exist and where they are to be found.

Most nursing professionals belong to a union, for example in Manufacturing, Science and Finance (MSF) there are three nursing sections – the CPHVA, the Community Psychiatric Nurses Association and the Nursery Nurses Network – and each has local representatives with access to advice from paid regional officials. Before you involve them you should take some first steps yourself (*see* Box 2.4).

MSF publishes detailed advice on many of these matters and it is always worth checking. Your local representative will have access to these publications.

The quality of working life

For the first time for many years, there is a recognition by the Department of Health that staff who are bullied, harassed, undervalued and not consulted are less productive and more likely to leave the NHS than staff who are not. The HR strategy states:

Box 2.4: Looking after yourself – get the procedures right

- Where there is any question of your individual *contract* of employment being amended deliberately or by default, then you should seek to clarify what has happened. For example, if your pay has dropped, check with payroll yourself why this is before involving anyone else
- Where there are any proposals to *change the way in which you or colleagues work* – workloads, skill mix, management structures, work base – then you should first seek clarification in writing as to what is proposed and why – and not agree to any changes before seeking advice
- Where you feel you are being *treated unfairly* then you should carefully record what is happening and its effects, and then take advice from your local representative
- Where you are concerned or told that you may be *disciplined*, you should take advice from a representative straight away to ensure the procedure is being followed
- Where you wish to complain about something – including about your grading – then you should take advice from your local representative before putting anything in writing

---

Box 2.5: Practice nurses

Most employees of NHS trusts and health authorities will find their employer has in place, on paper at least, many of the policies referred to above. There will normally be a recognition agreement for trade unions allowing trade unions to represent staff, meet with management, advise staff and be consulted on any proposed changes. There will generally be local representatives who have a right to be trained, have time off to advise and represent members, have some facilities (such as noticeboards, use of meeting rooms and telephones) and who management must meet when so requested.

This is not generally the case for practice nurses, other GP practice staff and for GPs who are not partners in the practice. The CPHVA will be publishing an employment rights handbook for practice nurses with detailed advice reflecting different circumstances for these colleagues.

The employment rights of practice staff will gradually improve and be harmonised with those of other NHS staff under the new HR strategy. Indeed it is likely that an increasing number of practice staff will become full NHS employees.

The best employers know that to obtain the best from their staff they must gain trust and treat them fairly and keep their promises to them. The link between quality service delivery and quality management of staff is at the heart of all good employment practice. There is now research evidence from the NHS itself which shows:

- poor staff management contributes to factors which damage the delicate infrastructure and networks that deliver patient care – and in turn exacerbates staff turnover, low morale and work-based stress and exhaustion.

Employers have a duty of care towards their staff. A breach of that duty has increasingly led staff to seek legal redress for bullying, harassment and excessive workloads. This duty parallels the duty for staff and nurse managers set out in the UKCC Code of Professional Conduct which states (para. 13) that every registered nurse midwife and health visitor must:

report to an appropriate person or authority where it appears that the health and safety of colleagues is at risk as such circumstances may compromise standards of practice and care.

The macho bullying ethos which pervades many NHS organisations is being directly challenged by this new approach. When Ministers state there will be 'zero tolerance for racism', that sends out a wider message about fair and equitable treatment. Amongst the initiatives staff should expect from their employers are:

- a serious development of family-friendly employment policies on job sharing, childcare, parental leave, flexible hours of work and maternity leave including rights on return from maternity leave

- a refusal to tolerate racism, sexism, homophobia, harassment and bullying of staff by colleagues, managers or the public

- a health improvement programme for staff linked to an audit of working practices to look at making working life less unhealthy – and therefore reducing absenteeism. This should include looking at the causes of stress – including excessive workloads, poor management, and a failure to value and nurture staff.

Crucial to an improvement in the quality of working life will be to create an organisation in which staff have real involvement in the development and management of the service and a real opportunity to develop their career and skills.

That means individual members of staff, and their union representatives, must be regarded as 'stakeholders' and partners in the new NHS, not, as often happens at present, as people who are told at the last minute of changes to their working lives and clinical practice.

Implications for management

Moves to improve the quality of working life should significantly benefit managers themselves since research repeatedly demonstrates that NHS managers are amongst the most stressed within the entire workforce.

The 'quality of working life agenda' should also help clarify management responsibilities to prevent the harassment, bullying, discrimination, overwork, alienation and stress many staff experience.

NHS organisations will need to be able to demonstrate that they have policies and procedures in place to prevent such risks and to deal effectively with them if they do occur.

Litigation is increasingly accompanying grievances taken through the internal procedures of NHS employers. Sensible management will want to be able to demonstrate that it has in place for quality of working life issues:

- measures to improve the quality of working life including published policies and procedures

- clear lines of accountability for such policies and procedures

- monitoring and evaluation of the most important ones

- clear means of complaint or redress for staff

- measures which draw upon the contribution of staff and involve them in developing better policies and monitoring the ones that exist – including involving trade unions.

Implications for employees

Changes in the law, and a changed attitude by the Department of Health, have created important rights and opportunities which should not be missed.

The recruitment and retention of nursing staff, together with the need to have a flexible workforce whose skills can change as the health service changes, means there is a widespread recognition that staff must be treated differently and treated better.

Where the right to be treated fairly and with respect is infringed it is essential that you challenge management. Where good policies exist it is important that staff understand them and use them. Where there are no policies or they are poorly observed, then staff must be pro-active in seeking to establish or to change them.

The best single way to do this is by becoming active in your trade union or professional organisation. Involvement in a trade union has several advantages over trying to tackle these issues on your own:

- a trade union has access to expert advice and will have come across your problem before somewhere else

- a trade union approach avoids individuals being singled out and victimised

- a trade union approach means there is a genuinely representative view of what staff feel about a particular problem

- a trade union has many local representatives who will know the best way to raise a problem locally and be aware of any similar local concerns.

Where an individual member of staff wishes to question or challenge a management decision, Box 2.6 summarises some simple recommended steps to follow to get the best results.

Box 2.6: Looking after yourself – first steps

1 Identify the problem by seeking clarification in writing of what management intentions are. Your local representative can assist with a letter

2 Find out what the local policies or agreements on this issue are

3 Find out what the local procedures for dealing with your problem are

4 Find out if anyone else has the same or similar concerns with grading, workloads, skill mix, training, and so on

5 Write down for yourself what you want to achieve by pursuing the issue

6 Talk to your local representative who can get additional expert advice if necessary and can then discuss with you how best to tackle the problem

Primary care groups

PCGs will not be the direct employers of anyone. They are sub-committees of the local health authority and any employees will be employed by the latter. That does not mean there are no HR implications arising from their work. There will be very significant HR issues and challenges arising from that role (*see* Box 2.7).

PCGs have clear governance arrangements. They are expected to:

- act as a united board and not act on behalf of any one group or profession (HSC 1998/139). In other words, GPs in particular are expected to place the goals of the PCGs (*see* Chapter 1) before their own practice or professional preferences

- act openly by having:

  - 'open and transparent processes'

  - 'regular communications with stakeholders'

Box 2.7: HR issues and PCGs

- In local NHS trusts   changes to working practices, priorities, skill mix, management arrangements, integration with practice staff, clinical governance

- In local GP practices   changes to working practices, priorities, skill mix, management arrangements, integration with trust staff, moves towards direct employment by local NHS trusts for some staff, clinical governance

- For the health authority   need to assume responsibility for HR issues and establish a local forum to discuss HR issues with trade unions and PCG board representatives, overall responsibility for clinical governance, employment arrangements for PCG staff and boards

---

- 'annual (and public) accountability agreements'

- 'clear and open clinical governance arrangements'

• promote the involvement of a wide range of staff in PCGs. This will most obviously be through the various local nursing forums which are intended to advise and support the nurse members of the PCG board

• work in partnership with other organisations – including NHS trusts. The relevant Guidance states:

> 'any unilateral action by any party . . . is unacceptable. It is the job of NHS Executive Regional Offices to performance manage this principle'.

This should mean that PCGs cannot, for example, unilaterally change service priorities and arrangements through commissioning services without first having discussed with the relevant trust whether the proposed changes are:

– appropriate
– feasible and safe
– subject to staff involvement and consultation

• take a lead on clinical governance – requiring careful consultation with staff and local employers.

HR issues will need to be integrated into the planning cycle of PCGs and referred to the health authority forum for joint consideration by management and the unions (*see* Box 2.8).

Who should get involved in influencing PCGs?

The health authority is responsible for the success of the PCG in implementing the HImP and its other priorities. It carries the can for its finances and for its success in implementing clinical governance. The chair of the PCG is the 'accountable officer' for the PCG board and is directly accountable to the chief executive of the health authority.

Box 2.8: PCG planning cycle and HR issues

Service priorities and resource allocation

lead to

Outline commissioning of services which should include discussions within the local nursing forum

followed by

Discussion with NHS trusts, GP practices and others providing services, as to the appropriateness, feasibility and consultation implications

including

Discussions in the joint negotiating committee of the trusts

Discussions in the health authority HR forum involving trades unions and professional organisations

leading to

Revised commissioning of services and budget setting

and

Formal discussions with trade unions on the trust joint negotiating committees and the health authority forums on the implications of any changes which include HR issues

accompanied by discussions with the Local Education and Training Consortia on the implications for future workforce planning

---

The local NHS trust management can seek to influence the PCG via discussions on the commissioning of services, particularly by spelling out the implications of any proposals for staffing, working arrangements, safe practice and consultation with staff and their trade unions.

The nursing staff employed by the local trust, and by local GP practices, can influence the PCG in three ways. Firstly, by participating in the local nursing forum they can influence professional and service decisions. Secondly, by ensuring that the best possible staff apply for the posts of nurse members of the PCG board. Thirdly, by having strong and effective trade unions they can use the health authority forum and the trust joint negotiating committee to ensure they are consulted on HR issues arising from PCG proposals.

Box 2.9 shows how these opportunities all fit together.

Box 2.9: Influencing the PCG

1   Nurse members of PCG boards are there to ensure a *nursing* perspective in the commissioning of services and other activities of the PCG board.

   They are *not* there to represent *nurses*.

2   The *local nursing forum* (or committee) is there to support and advise the nurse members of the PCG board in that *nursing* perspective.

   They are *not* there to represent *nurses*. They should not get involved in matters that involve the representation of nurses in any matters relating to their employment. Nor is it their job to replace trust managers and staff who lead on professional issues.

3   The *Trust Joint Negotiating Committee* is there to negotiate with trust management and be consulted by trust management on all aspects of HR, employment and such other issues agreed locally to be legitimate business for the committee. In the spirit of Social Partnership that would certainly include training, clinical governance, equal opportunities, the management of change, professional and managerial structures, skill mix and so on.

4   The *health authority forum* is there to ensure that there is a body for trade unions to be consulted on and negotiated with, as appropriate, on HR issues arising from PCGs covered by any one health authority. Its role is to ensure consistent standards for trust employees and to avoid duplication of effort.

   Its membership is to be determined locally by agreement between health authorities and trade unions.

5   Membership of all four bodies should be facilitated and supported by trusts and health authorities with appropriate paid cover, time off, training and facilities.

The NHS Executive Guidance makes it clear that staff involvement in these activities should be supported and funded:

NHS trusts and other employers should ensure that health professionals are encouraged and facilitated to take part in the work of PCGs

and

the travelling and other personal expenses of professionals not employed by a health authority but involved in working with

PCGs should, where appropriate and possible, be recognised and reimbursed accordingly from the management resources available to that health authority or group.

The remuneration for PCG board members provides for the same payment regardless of the profession of the board member. There is also provision for payment for locum arrangements to GPs and nurses who require cover for their clinical work whilst on PCG business.

It then goes on to set out a clear framework within which PCG HR issues should be discussed:

Health authorities should consider establishing a forum which could helpfully provide a useful vehicle to discuss human resource and organisational development issues for community nurses and provide a means to co-ordinate the development of primary care groups in that area.

Box 2.10: How it should all hang together

The future workforce needs driven by changing services

plus

labour shortages in areas of health professional services plus capped resources

means

pressure to redesign workforce plus skill mix/multi-skilling

which needs

a new pay system to allow for more flexible working and which is equal pay proofed

alongside

a clinical governance structure with improved training and continuing professional development (CPD)

which together with

a Health Improvement Programme for staff

and

a management which has the capacity and skills to deliver a new approach to managing change

will be

consulted on and negotiated on from start to finish by truly representative trade unions or, if they do not meet this criterion, by other forms of staff organisation

all of which will help to deliver

the right numbers of the right mixture of staff with the right skills at the right time within available resources

3

Planning and commissioning

Denise Hagel

The aim of this chapter is to assess the impact of changes to the planning and commissioning of health services in the 'new NHS'. The overall effect – bringing planning and commissioning down to primary care group (PCG) level – is to bring all health visitors and community nurses much closer to the processes involved. Regardless of whether they have a seat on the PCG board or not, all community practitioners will be involved in decisions which decide the amount, quality and structure of health services for their local community. Their information and local knowledge will be essential for planning, and their public health skills will be invaluable for the new community-wide approach. PCGs represent the best opportunity in the history of health service reform for community nurses to use their unique knowledge and skills to improve the health of communities.

Review of the changes

The changes to planning and commissioning in *The New NHS* have been described in Chapter 1. In summary:

- the term 'commissioning' replaces 'purchasing', reflecting the new emphasis on collaboration rather than competition
- the commissioners will eventually be only PCGs, although initially health authorities will continue to commission some services, agreed with the PCG boards; full PCG commissioning will happen incrementally, as the groups develop capability
- 'commissioning' requires the negotiation of longer-term (3- or 5-year) funding and service agreements with trusts
- eventually primary care trusts (PCTs) will employ community nurses (*see* Chapter 6) but at present commissioning includes service agreements with community or combined trusts for community nursing and health visiting services
- services commissioned by PCGs have to be both responsive to the needs of the local community and in line with the local Health Improvement Programme (HImP; *see* Box 3.1)
- the funding available to the PCG for commissioning services is cash-limited.

Box 3.1: A reminder: the Health Improvement Programme

The HImP:

- is a local strategy for improving health and healthcare
- is developed by the health authority in consultation with local authorities, local trusts, PCGs, other professionals such as dentists and pharmacists, the public and other partner organisations
- covers a three-year period, and part is updated each year
- covers the main health needs and healthcare requirements of the local people, and the investment required in local health services to meet these needs
- includes targets from *Our Healthier Nation* and the National Service Frameworks for Assessing Performance
- is binding on the PCGs and PCTs in the area

Box 3.2: Collaboration: a definition

Collaboration – 'to work jointly with'

General issues arising from the changes

These changes raise a number of key issues for everyone involved in PCGs, as well as specific issues for community practitioners.

Collaboration

The word 'collaboration' appears frequently in the White Paper *The New NHS* as a new way of working following the dismantling of the internal market (*see* Box 3.2). But collaboration will not happen automatically in primary care, and collaboration across agencies and sectors is even more difficult to put into practice. The rhetoric of a new way of working will need practical systems of co-operation and communication to make it happen. There are existing initiatives and capabilities on which PCGs could build:

- many health visitors and community nurses have valuable experience of working across agencies, and developing networks and contacts in order to achieve very real objectives in the care of their clients. These skills and networks need to be linked in to the planning and commissioning work of the PCGs, so that they build on existing relationships rather than trying to start new networks from an artificial 'clean sheet'

- integrated nursing teams exist in many areas, combining all community nurses, including practice nurses, and health visitors, into one, usually self-managed team (*see* Box 3.3). These teams could be set up in every practice in a PCG, and linked across the PCG, to create a strong community nursing voice to feed into the board through the nurse board members.

Box 3.3: Integrated nursing teams: characteristics and benefits

Integrated teams have been defined as a 'team of community-based nurses from different disciplines working in a primary care setting, pooling their skills, knowledge and abilities to provide the most effective care for the practice population it covers'.*

The important principles underlying it are that:

- it has common values, aims and objectives

- it is nurse-led

- it develops in response to defined areas of need within the population

- it has clear lines of communication and accountability, increased authority and autonomy.

Working as an integrated nursing team does not require nurses to step directly into each other's role; rather it requires flexibility, with a reduction in role overlap. It does not create a generic nurse but rather builds on and develops individual's specialities.

Figure 3.1 shows where there can be areas of role overlap. The competences in health needs assessment, service development, clinical governance, educational needs assessment etc., would be expected from a qualified community nurse specialist.

*Black S and Hagel D (1996) Developing an integrated nursing team approach. *Health Visitor.* **69.**

Input to the Health Improvement Programme

PCGs' input to the local HImP also needs to be identified in real terms. If the programme is to be genuinely linked to local needs and priorities, then individual PCGs will need the capacity to take a public health approach to the needs of their local community (*see* Box 3.4). This is something which individual GP practices have not traditionally been required to do, and will represent one of the biggest changes, and challenges, for the PCGs. GPs, who form the majority on PCG boards, need to acquire this new perspective in

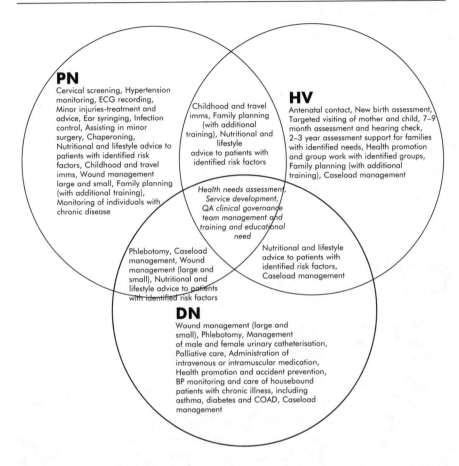

PN
Cervical screening, Hypertension monitoring, ECG recording, Minor injuries-treatment and advice, Ear syringing, Infection control, Assisting in minor surgery, Chaperoning, Nutritional and lifestyle advice to patients with identified risk factors, Childhood and travel imms, Wound management large and small, Family planning (with additional training), Monitoring of individuals with chronic disease

Childhood and travel imms, Family planning (with additional training), Nutritional and lifestyle advice to patients with identified risk factors

HV
Antenatal contact, New birth assessment, Targeted visiting of mother and child, 7–9 month assessment and hearing check, 2–3 year assessment support for families with identified needs, Health promotion and group work with identified groups, Family planning (with additional training), Caseload management

Health needs assessment, Service development, QA clinical governance team management and training and educational need

Phlebotomy, Caseload management, Wound management (large and small), Nutritional and lifestyle advice to patients with identified risk factors

Nutritional and lifestyle advice to patients with identified risk factors, Caseload management

DN
Wound management (large and small), Phlebotomy, Management of male and female urinary catheterisation, Palliative care, Administration of intravenous or intramuscular medication, Health promotion and accident prevention, BP monitoring and care of housebound patients with chronic illness, including asthma, diabetes and COAD, Caseload management

Figure 3.1   Areas of role overlap.

order for the PCG to fulfil its obligations to identify and meet community health needs. Again, existing skills and mechanisms need to be harnessed to the new way of working, in addition to the development of new capabilities.

- Profiling and needs assessment, and the discrimination between competing priorities, are skills already possessed by members of the primary healthcare team, in particular by health visitors. PCGs will need to make time and opportunities for individual practitioners to carry out these activities, and to convert the rich

Box 3.4: Characteristics of a public health approach

- An approach which is multi-disciplinary not generalist
- A concern with health and the whole person
- A concern with people which is not confined to their status as patients
- A concern with groups of people and communities
- An interest in prevention and early diagnosis of disease
- Responsive to the views of patients, carers and communities
- A longer-term strategic view with a population focus
- Needs assessment of groups and populations
- Works through others (to manage change)

data they already possess into meaningful and useable information. Mechanisms need to be set up so that this work is fed into the planning and commissioning timetable of the board.

- Different models of health visiting already exist, offering a public health practitioner role complementary to the family support role. While the latter still takes a public health approach by working with individuals in their communities, the public health practitioner focuses on community and public health issues (*see* Box 3.5).

- Currently, non-medical public health workers do exist, but have very limited career opportunities, and generally work under medical public health hierarchies. There is an urgent need to develop a robust and autonomous public heath career structure for non-medical practitioners.

- All nurses have recently been encouraged to identify and strengthen the public health aspects of their role (SNMAC, 1995). Some community nurses have traditionally focused on a caseload of individual patients and disregarded the population at large. This needs to change so that all community practitioners in a PCG recognise the whole population of the local

---

Box 3.5: A public health model of health visiting

- Neighbourhood or patch (PCG)-based
- Does not carry 0–5 caseload
- Acts as a public health resource to primary care
- Provides the link between public health departments and primary care
- Compiles Community Health Profiles which identify health needs of the community to support planning and commissioning of services
- Co-ordinates and draws together plans of all agencies for improving health in the neighbourhood
- Delegated authority from health authority to support and co-ordinate cross-sectoral input to HImP
- Engages in and supports inter-sectoral collaboration and community participation

---

community as the focus of their work, and consciously develop the public health approach described by SNMAC (*see* Box 3.6).

Preparation for board responsibilities

The PCG boards (*see* Table 3.1) are made up of a range of different professional and lay people, who have not previously worked

Table 3.1 A reminder: composition of the PCG board

Designation	Number of representatives	Method of selection
GPs	4–7	Election
Community nurses	1–2	Election or selection
Social services officer	1	Nomination by local authority
Lay member	1	Nomination by health authority
Health authority non-executive	1	Nominated by HA
PCG chief officer (ex-officio, non-voting member)	1	Appointed by the board

Box 3.6: Characteristics of a public health approach to nursing, from 'Making It Happen' (SNMAC, 1995)

SNMAC agrees that '*public health in nursing, midwifery and health visiting practice is about commissioning health services and providing professional care through organised collaboration in the NHS and society, to protect and promote health and well-being, prolong life and prevent ill health in local communities, groups and populations*'.

SNMAC emphasises that the contribution of the nursing professions to public health is underlined by the following concepts:

- use of *public health approaches*, perspectives and objectives in health commissioning and provision of services. In general, the identification of health needs and desired outcomes, agreement on the most effective and acceptable action and evaluation, including user perspectives throughout, are typical features of a public health approach
- a knowledge of *population health needs* even when caring for individuals. The population may range from identified client groups to whole communities or large geographical areas
- an emphasis on collective and collaborative action
- a recognition of people as members of groups, not only as individuals
- a *public health perspective* which anchors clinical and non-clinical care in the social, organisational and policy aspects of health development
- a focus on health promotion, in enabling people to increase control over and improve their health, combined with preventing disease.

together. They will undertake the planning and commissioning which was previously the remit of the health authority or fundholders. Preparing investment plans, setting up funding and service agreements, allocating cash-limited development monies and monitoring the quality of secondary care services are new roles for most of the PCG board members. They will not be able to undertake these activities without intensive preparation in the form of training, work shadowing, coaching or tandem working with health authority managers. Community nurses and health visitors on boards will need to be given time and opportunities to prepare in this way if they are to be effective members of the board. Some of the specific competencies which will be needed on the board include:

- strategic planning
- profiling and health needs assessment
- service specification and commissioning
- understanding of secondary care services
- service quality specification and monitoring
- resource prioritisation
- financial management and planning
- workforce planning.

It will not be necessary for every member of the board to have all the competencies needed. Each member brings different skills and competencies, and additional expertise can be co-opted on to the board as necessary. However, the board is collectively responsible for its planning and commissioning decisions, and community practitioners on the board will need to be sufficiently aware of the key issues in each area to enable them to participate in corporate decision making. The board as a whole will undergo considerable organisational development in its first few years of existence, and may need to arrange expert coaching to do this.

Resource allocation

One of the roles of the PCG board will be the allocation of cash-limited resources for the funding of healthcare. Boards will be making the decisions, previously made by health authorities, about which services or treatments can and cannot be funded (*see* Box 3.7). This has several significant consequences:

- it involves community practitioners for the first time in the rationing of healthcare
- as well as participating in the financial decisions, community practitioners will be involved in ethical decisions about the

---

Box 3.7: Examples of rationing decisions made by health authorities

On basis of cost:
Availability of infertility treatments on NHS
Gender re-assignment

On basis of judgement about evidence of effectiveness:
Availability of interferon treatment for multiple sclerosis
Universal availability of new anti-dementia treatment
Homeopathic/alternative therapies

On basis of perceived cost–benefit ratio:
Additional cycles of treatment for relapsed patient with leukaemia

---

availability of treatments through the NHS

- rationing decisions will require sophisticated and informed appraisal of the evidence of clinical effectiveness, cost-effectiveness and population health gain

- the board, and all professionals working in the PCG, will have to deal with any conflict between the need or demand for services and the funding available to supply them

- PCGs are required to have open meetings and consult with members of the community which they serve. Decisions about investment or disinvestment in services will be subject to close local scrutiny, and practitioners will have to be able on occasions to explain decisions directly to their patients or clients.

The cash-limited budget

The unified, cash-limited budgets allocated to PCGs change the way in which spending on healthcare has historically been managed (*see* Figure 3.2). The most significant aspect of the unification of budgets is the capacity to 'move money around' between areas that would previously have been managed separately. This has the advantage of flexibility, enabling prudence in one area to enable additional spending in another. The disadvantage is that increased spending incurred in one area reduces the funding available for spending in another.

Previously:

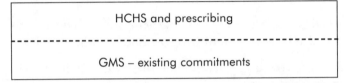

Hospital and community health services	General Medical Services (cash-limited): staff, premises, computers	General Medical Services (non-cash-limited): prescribing

Now:

HCHS and prescribing
- -
GMS – existing commitments

Figure 3.2   A reminder: changes to funding in the new NHS.

The most significant aspects of this new budgetary system are:

- community practitioners can directly influence decisions about spending priorities for the first time, through their members on the PCG board. At this local level, for example, district nurses could produce a costed plan for their population to demonstrate that money spent on training, equipment and consumables for compression bandaging for venous leg ulcers could save the PCG the costs of longer-term, less effective treatment, including additional visits by nursing staff

- as the PCGs have responsibility for developing community nursing and the budget for practice staffing, as well as the capacity to move money around between areas of spending, nurses in integrated teams are in an ideal position to advise the board on staffing and skills requirements. The unified budget, and the 'corporate' overview of all the practices in the PCG, will allow more flexible and innovative patterns of working to be tried out.

Summary of general issues in planning and commissioning

The new arrangements in PCGs for planning and commissioning of healthcare and health services should mean:

• community practitioners' collaborative ways of working will become the norm

• community practitioners' 'grass roots' information will be able to influence the Health Improvement Programmes for the district

• different models of working, particularly of public health work, will become more common

• PCGs will develop a public health approach, in contrast to the traditional individual practice approach

• all community nurses will have enhanced public health roles

• many community practitioners will develop new skills and competencies

• PCG board members will take on new responsibilities, including for difficult ethical and financial decisions

• community practitioners will have more influence on how local health service money is spent

• they will also be able to influence the development of community nursing in their PCG.

Specific issues for community practitioners

In addition to the general issues arising from the new commissioning agenda, there are some issues which are specific to, or of particular interest to, community practitioners. These are:

• the need for skills acquisition for *all* community nurses

• the potential for conflicts of interest between PCG and trust

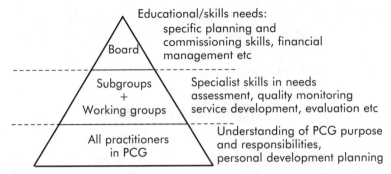

Figure 3.3   Skills and education needs of practitioners in PCGs.

- the necessity for unification of community nursing

- the role of the nurses on the PCG board

- the need for strong nursing leadership at district level and above

- clinical governance and quality issues for nurses in PCGs

- the PCGs' role in developing community nursing.

Skills for all

There is clearly a need for the acquisition of particular skills by nurses on the boards of PCGs. These have already been listed, and include strategic planning, health needs assessment and service planning, among others. But there is also a need for all community practitioners to develop an understanding of the key issues, and for many of them to acquire particular skills such as quality assessment, audit, service evaluation or patient advocacy. This is because many of the nurses, health visitors and other professionals in a PCG will become involved in subgroups of the board, examining and advising on particular issues. These might be as broad as 'clinical governance', or as specific as a review of maternity services or the impact of increased nurse prescribing. Even those practitioners who choose not to, or do not have the opportunity to, contribute to any of the working groups will need to be aware of the issues being tackled, and the developments in their

PCG which may affect them and their clients (*see* Figure 3.3). As the PCGs mature, and time passes, the current board members will move on and need to be replaced by new appointees. It is essential that there are community nurses with the knowledge and awareness to take over places on the board in the future.

The potential conflict of interest

Community practitioners who are employed by a trust, and who have worked for a fundholding practice in the past, will be aware of the potential for conflict between their trust employer and the practice or group of practices for whom they provide nursing or health visiting services. Trusts work on a larger scale, with management systems, policies and procedures applying across a range of different working situations; the individual practice may have wanted to use their purchasing freedom to try out new methods of working, or to tailor a service to their population.

The same potential for conflict exists in a PCG. With a budget for services for around 100 000 people, and the staffing resource attached to, or employed by, a relatively large group of practices, it is inevitable that PCGs will want to try different methods of maximising the community nursing input. This could include individual practitioners working across practices, or the use of different models of service delivery, or a move to much larger integrated teams.

Trusts will have to combine new degrees of flexibility with the provision of robust staff support when necessary. Practitioners need to recognise the significance of the difference between the inclusive PCGs and the old, individual fundholders. Opting out, or simply lying low, is not possible: all practitioners are members of a PCG, which is a smaller and more transparent organisation than a trust and, unlike a fundholding practice, the standard model in primary care. Every practitioner needs to be prepared to adapt to new ways of working, where these may enhance the provision of a skilled, seamless and comprehensive service to the population. They also need to be prepared to assess, professionally and objectively, proposals by their PCG for changes to existing patterns of provision. Where they believe that these will harm, or fail to improve, service provision, they need to be prepared to make proper representation to that effect to the PCG board, through the community nurse members or other mechanisms established by the PCG. A trust's staff may be scattered amongst a number of different PCGs and trust managers will not necessarily be able to take on that role for their staff.

The unification of community nursing

The changes in *The New NHS* will not produce a generic community nurse. But they do treat community nurses – including school nurses, midwives and health visitors, who may not always describe themselves by that label – as one group. Places on PCG boards are open to any nurse working in primary care, and, with two places on the board, it is unlikely that any PCG has the full range of specialisms working at board level, even if additional nurse members have been co-opted.

In this situation, it is essential that all community nurses, whether trust-employed or practice-employed, also regard themselves as one unified group of professionals. The development of integrated nursing teams has begun this process in many areas, helping to overcome the obstacles of different employers and separate lines of management. Now all community nurses in an area work for the same 'organisation' (the PCG) and the same population (the community served by the PCG). They only need to change their historically divided perceptions of themselves to become part of a much larger, more truly integrated and potentially powerful group of nurses, with direct access to the planning and commissioning decision makers.

Leadership across PCGs

Within each PCG, the unified nurses can expect to contribute to plans for both patient services and for the development of nursing in the group. But across a number of PCGs, it is essential that there is strong, effective nursing leadership at health authority level. This will contribute to the performance management of the PCGs in general, and to strategic planning regarding nursing services in particular.

Clinical governance and community practitioners

This topic is explored in more detail in Chapter 4. It is a major issue for community nurses, as providers of the great majority of the assessment, treatment, care and advocacy for the PCG's population. The elements of clinical governance, which include audit, risk assessment, health and safety, continuing professional development, standard setting and implementation of best practice, are all integral parts of good nursing practice. For the first time, however, these elements will be systematically scrutinised and form the basis of an annual accountability report from the PCG board to the chief executive of the health authority. The opportunities for practitioners to focus the board's attention on quality rather than finance, and to highlight and disseminate excellence in their practice, need to be grasped and exploited.

The role of nurses on the board

The guidance on the setting up of PCGs made it clear that the role of the nurses on the board was to bring a community nursing perspective to PCG decision making, not to represent a particular group of nurses, or even nursing as a whole. In addition, the PCGs are new bodies, the boards are new groups of people who have not formerly worked together, and the role of the board in planning and commissioning at community level is yet to be fully developed. Given this wide brief and lack of any comparable precedent, it is inevitably going to take some time for nurse board members to develop a clear view of their role. They will need to be prepared to be adaptable and to actively shape the role, rather than allow it to be minimalised by competing pressures from other board members. They will also need the active and objective support of other community practitioners in the PCG. With a wide range of new skills to acquire, a place to establish at the board table and a heavy agenda of PCG business, the nurse members will be looking to subgroups and working groups to advise, assist and support them. In the early years of PCGs, with the political and professional spotlight on them, it is absolutely essential that nurses are seen to contribute effectively to successful planning and commissioning.

The PCG's role in developing community nursing

Each PCG will produce a primary care investment plan which includes plans for the development of community nursing. This raises a number of issues of concern to community nurses:

- the inevitable medical influence, from the GP-dominated PCG board, on the development of nursing

- the potential conflict between trusts employing nurses and the PCG's plans, between the practitioners themselves and the PCG's plans, and between the professional and statutory bodies in nursing and the PCG's plans

- the lack of expertise in, or understanding of, nursing by the GP majority on boards

- the absence of links between PCGs and the educational consortia, which deploy the funding for non-medical education and training

- the unresolved professional issues of skill- and grade-mix, and the place of newer developments such as nurse practitioners and the proposed nurse consultants, which may be included in the plans

- the need for more sophisticated commissioning of nursing and health visiting services, focusing on outcomes to be achieved rather than tasks to be undertaken.

What community practitioners can do ...

The major work of the PCGs cannot be achieved by the boards working in isolation. They do not have the time or the full range of expertise, and they need to consult with all practitioners working in the PCG, as well as with formal subgroups or working groups. Equally, every practitioner working in a PCG has to take responsibility for their part in helping the organisation to plan and commission health services, and to develop the internal capability of the PCG itself. Community practitioners have much of the necessary experience, and many of the necessary skills, already. So what can community practitioners do, in practical terms, to contribute:

... to systems for collaborative working?

- ensure that they understand integrated nursing teams, can identify working examples and describe the advantages to the PCG board if necessary

- get together in their own practice-based or larger team to put the principles of integrated working into practice

- discuss the advantages of appointing a dedicated public health worker, in addition to the public health work of team members, to act as a resource to both teams and the board

- develop links with both the local health authority and local authority social services department by getting to know the relevant representatives on their PCG board.

... to facilitate their PCG's contribution to the HImP?

- collate existing profile data from members of each practice-based team

- think about how it could be presented as a single profile of the whole PCG area

- offer the information, in accessible form, to the board, through the nurse members

- establish mechanisms for a two-way dialogue between the board and practitioners in the PCG, for example, through meetings with board members, attendance at open board meetings, a PCG-wide newsletter or a combination of these and other methods.

... about developing the PCG's public health capability?

- make existing public health knowledge and skills available to teams and the PCG board

- identify public health projects, posts or work already underway within the PCG, and make them known to the board

- discuss the development of a public health approach with the local authority representative on the board, to link in with local authority environmental and housing initiatives

... about skills acquisition for individuals and the PCG organisation?

- agree a link person in each primary healthcare team to co-ordinate skills audits and requests for training

- identify a link to the education consortium, possibly through the nurse adviser at health authority level

- get a copy of the organisational development toolkit available from the NHS Executive, and use it

- use personal development plans to identify personal knowledge or development needs, and collate at team level for the link person to take forward; aim to fill gaps in team knowledge or skills, rather than equip every member with every skill

- agree an educational strategy for the team, involving both experiential and formal learning

- lobby the PCG board for joint training between different professions whenever possible, and in particular on planning and commissioning topics

- arrange sessions with individuals, such as current or former health authority commissioning managers or finance managers, to provide broad understanding of the terms and issues for the team members.

... about tackling rationing issues?

- discuss, within and between teams, the ethical and professional issues involved, and personal strategies for coping with pressure or censure from patients

- establish a dialogue with the board about involving and informing the public: cite examples of partnership decision making, such as maternity services liaison committees

- get to know the lay person on the PCG board, and their links with the community

... about the financial issues?

- ensure that all practitioners understand the meaning of the terms used, and their significance: produce a glossary in a PCG newsletter

- ask the board, through the nurse members, for details of real information: the total allocation to the PCG, whether over-spends from the health authority have been carried forward into the PCG budget, what the historical spending for the practices in the PCG has been

- ask about the primary care investment plan, which will include new nursing posts or changes to existing posts: put a summary in the PCG newsletter.

... about clinical governance?

- find out who is the PCG lead for clinical governance – it could be doctor or a nurse

- suggest that the post alternates between the two professions, or is held jointly

- find out who is responsible for clinical governance in individual practices, and arrange sharing of information

- inform the board of existing mechanisms or groups which have something to contribute, such as journal clubs, research groups, audit group members

- ask the clinical governance lead which performance indicators are to be used for the PCG, and review the nursing contribution to each.

... about the role of the nurse on the board?

- arrange for the team to meet with the board nurse members at regular intervals
- decide how information is to be passed between the board members and other practitioners between meetings
- agree what support and input the board members can expect from other practitioners in the group
- ask for reports from each PCG board meeting from the nurse members.

... about the PCG's role in developing community nursing?

- collect information on and examples of different models of community nursing and health visiting, and make them available to the board
- identify the evidence of effectiveness of different nursing models, and their application to particular health or community needs
- set up mechanisms for two-way dialogue with the board about nursing issues, through the nurse members and other routes
- find examples of services or areas where community nursing is commissioned on the basis of outcomes rather than inputs, and present to the board.

Summary

- *The New NHS* brings a major change in emphasis and approach to the planning and commissioning of health services. Collaboration replaces competition, and the commissioners will eventually be solely the PCG boards, made up principally of GPs and community nurses.

- These changes will have a direct impact on all community practitioners, whether or not they are members of a PCG board.

- Community practitioners need to use the collaborative power they already have as a result of their unique information base about communities and their needs, and their existing public health, community development and consumer advocacy skills.

- PCGs need to be encouraged to develop new ways of commissioning: for outcomes rather than tasks, with new service agreement currencies based on health gain rather than numbers of contacts.

- Community practitioners need to recognise the new agenda will affect everyone, and that everyone should expect to change practice in the new NHS.

4

Clinical governance

Thelma Sackman

What is clinical governance? Is it new, or is it a new title for current activities? I believe that clinical governance is an all-embracing statement, which aims to identify and implement high quality healthcare services. To introduce clinical governance, the Government launched in December 1997, *The New NHS: modern, dependable*. This stated:

> Professional and Statutory Bodies have a vital role in setting and prioritising standards; but shifting the focus towards quality will also require practitioners to accept responsibility for developing and maintaining standards within their local NHS organisations. For this reason the Government will require every NHS Trust to embrace the concept of 'Clinical Governance' so that quality is at the core both of their responsibility or organisation and of each of their staff as individual professionals.

'Clinical governance is inclusive, there can be no opting out.' HSC 1998/139 *Developing Primary Care Groups* goes on to stress that the whole clinical governance process should aim to be reflective and supportive for doctors, nurses and other health professionals operating within primary care groups (PCGs) (*see* Box 4.1).

Box 4.1: Definition of clinical governance

'Clinical governance can be defined as a framework through which NHS organisations are accountable for continuously improving the quality of their services and safeguarding high standards of care by creating an environment in which excellence in clinical care will flourish.'

These statements need to be unpicked to identify what they mean for practitioners.

- Are practitioners going to have to change practice?
- Are they going to have to spend more time on bureaucratic processes?
- Can clinical governance be embraced within the concept of everyday practice?

It is important to identify what is happening in practice and what can be done to embrace the principles of clinical governance. This chapter will identify some of the key elements of clinical governance that practitioners need to consider and will reflect clinical practice with a particular focus on community practitioners.

Key elements

The key elements of clinical governance are:

- clinical effectiveness
- clinical audit
- professional self-regulation
- lifelong learning
- clinical risk management
- policies, procedures and protocols

- partnerships in practice

- information technology.

Clinical effectiveness

There are a number of definitions for clinical effectiveness, however, the main emphasis is about getting the appropriate and relevant care to a patient or client at the right time. At its conference in October 1998 the CPHVA launched a *Clinical Effectiveness Information Pack*. This pack identifies the key features of clinical effectiveness interventions:

- they are based on the best evidence available

- the evidence is implemented in practice within a systematic framework of monitoring and review

- they achieve the intended process of care and health outcomes based on clients' needs.

The NHS Executive also launched a pack in 1998 called *Achieving Effective Practice: a clinical effectiveness and research information pack for nurses, midwives and health visitors*. These two packs will help practitioners to embrace the concept of clinically effective practice, as they give valuable information and case studies regarding clinically effective practice. In outline, the process of clinically effective practice is a staged approach:

Stage 1 – Develop an understanding of clinical effectiveness.

Stage 2 – Identify current practice and question whether this practice is evidence-based and meeting the patients'/clients' needs.

Stage 3 – Identify relevant research, critically review the information and evaluate current practice against this evidence.

Stage 4 – Change practice where appropriate to accommodate your findings.

Stage 5 – Re-evaluate, audit and review practice.

What should community practitioners do about clinical effectiveness? Some possibilities are:

- work in professional groups to enable those with particular interest to lead on a clinical effectiveness topic

- link these topics to standards in practice

- use the information in the development of clinical protocols and clinical guidelines

- develop a programme of work locally to embrace the clinical effectiveness agenda and influence the priorities for action at PCG, NHS trust and health authority level.

Clinical audit

Clinical audit is an activity that enables practitioners to examine the effectiveness of their services (*see* Box 4.2). It will become a critical tool in the management of performance against agreed standards. All clinicians will be expected to undertake and participate in clinical audit programmes, particularly looking at the New National Performance Framework. These will be focusing on six themes:

- health improvement

- fair access to service

- effective delivery of appropriate healthcare

- efficiency

- patient and carer experiences

- outcomes of NHS care.

Box 4.2: Clinical audit

'A clinically led initiative which seeks to improve the quality and outcome of patient care through structured peer review, whereby clinicians examine their practice and results against agreed explicit standards and modify their practice where indicated.'

(NHS Executive 1996 – Clinical Audit in the NHS. Using Clinical Audit in the NHS: A Position Statement)

Box 4.3: The Commission for Health Improvement

The Commission's core function will be to:

- provide national leadership to develop and disseminate clinical governance principles

- independently scrutinise local clinical governance arrangements to support, promote and deliver high quality services, through a rolling programme of local reviews of service providers

- undertake a programme of service reviews to monitor national implementation of National Service Frameworks, and review progress locally on implementation of these Frameworks and NICE guidance

- help the NHS identify and tackle serious or persistent clinical problems. The Commission will have the capacity for rapid investigation and intervention to help put these right

- over time, increasingly take on responsibility for overseeing and assisting with external incident inquiries

---

It is essential that the audit cycle works within the clinical effectiveness framework to ensure research-based practice. The Government will be setting up the Commission for Health Improvement (CHI) which will be monitoring the quality of services in the NHS and will wish to see the systems that organisations and practitioners have in place to review and where necessary improve patient care (*see* Box 4.3).

Documenting the work and the outcomes will be prerequisite, as will evidence of any changes in clinical practice and service delivery. Clinical audit is an essential tool for community practitioners to understand and to use, as it will help identify resources required to enhance the quality of services. An example of clinical audit is shown in Box 4.4.

Clinical effectiveness and clinical audit are part of the governance agenda. Other important issues include professional self-regulation and lifelong learning, which aim to strengthen and build on good practice, and to ensure that poor performance is dealt with quickly and appropriately.

Box 4.4: An example of clinical audit

Improving breastfeeding information and support.

This project involved the implementation of a standard practice for health visitors on the provision of breastfeeding information and support.

Why was the audit needed? Discussion in the North East Fife professional focus group prompted health visitors in the district to explore their attitudes and knowledge about breastfeeding. It was decided that the health visitors as a group should tackle conflicting advice given by members of their own profession. An initial audit was needed to describe and review the current situation.

How was the project carried out? Stringent criteria for successful breastfeeding were set, and a baseline audit carried out by all the health visitors in the district. A standard was then set, using the Donabedian process. The standard statement was that: 'All women who wish to breastfeed will be given all appropriate information and support', and structure, process and outcome criteria were devised. All advice would be based on a knowledge of normal feeding patterns and current research on breastfeeding. A year after the implementation of the standard a further audit was carried out to assess whether the standard of practice was being met; to identify reasons if the standard was not being met; to identify amendments required, and to collect statistics on successful breastfeeders, according to the set criteria.

Results of the project and changes initiated: the results of the second audit showed an increase of almost 10% in successful breast-feeding. Although the audit in the following year showed a drop of 7%, this still represented an overall increase from the baseline figure. The audit of the standard highlighted areas of need for health visitor training and professional development, access to recent publications, knowledge of local agencies to support breastfeeding and also the need for a breastfeeding advisory leaflet. Action was taken in all these areas as a result of the audit project.

Professional self-regulation

In *A First Class Service* the Government identified that professional self-regulation is an essential part of quality patient services. The UKCC has responsibility for developing the standards for education, training and professional conduct for all registered nurses, midwives and health visitors. The main responsibility of the UKCC is to protect the interests of the public. The Code of

Professional Conduct was drawn up under the powers of the Nurses, Midwives and Health Visitors Act 1979 to give advice to registered practitioners. All registered practitioners need to reflect on the meaning of the code and the personal and professional accountability that is contained within the 16 clauses.

To strengthen the role of the professional self-regulation bodies they need to be:

- more open

- more publicly accountable and

- be able to respond to change.

What community practitioners need to do is:

- maintain professional registration through continued professional development which addresses current clinical practice. The UKCC's post-registration, education and practice (PREP) programme requires nurses, midwives and health visitors to maintain and improve standards of care and promote higher standards of practice

- maintain a personal professional profile recording all aspects of professional development. These profiles will also be extremely helpful for practitioners when they are looking at their lifelong learning requirements and fits well with the statement set out in *A First Class Service* (*see* Box 4.5).

Lifelong learning (LLL)/continuous professional development (CPD)

Through PREP, nurses, midwives and health visitors have to undertake a minimum of five days or equivalent study activities every three years to enable them to renew and maintain their registration. Lifelong learning is essential to improve quality and to keep pace with the fast changing evidence, knowledge and expertise associated with health and healthcare.

Box 4.5: Investing in lifelong learning

We will work with professional and education bodies, staff representative organisations and NHS employers to explore a range of
practical issues including:

- the role of monitoring, peer review and appraisal
- the role of new technology and distance learning in maximising
  learning opportunities and customising the process
- how the expertise of professional and statutory bodies can best
  support local CPD, within the context of clinical governance
- the educational infrastructure required to identify and meet CPD
  needs

Community practitioners will be required to:

- write their own personal development plans, taking into consideration the needs of the service being provided as well as
  professional issues
- do this in discussion with local colleagues
- identify how their personal development plans are to be implemented
- influence local training initiatives
- identify who will co-ordinate the training programmes
- establish how priorities will be assessed.

The NHS organisations need to ensure that the continuous professional development programmes support not only those issues
identified in personal development plans, but also the locally and
nationally agreed priorities. If the Government emphasis is on
poverty, deprivation, social exclusion, parenting skills, etc., then
the education, training and development schemes must be in place
locally to meet these initiatives. Meeting major Government
targets requires partnership between practitioners, NHS organisations and education providers.

Lifelong learning must also reflect the outcomes of clinical audit, evidence-based practice and skills developments. There has to be a major investment both personally and organisationally to ensure that practitioners are kept up to date and are competent to practice.

Some practitioners are already investing a significant amount of their personal and organisational time on development. This may include:

- reflective practice

- clinical supervision

- peer review

- education courses

- alternative experience

- skills development

- research

- audit.

Nurses, midwives and health visitors have a duty of care, and lifelong learning will help maintain standards of care and in some instances advance practice.

Clinical risk management (see Box 4.6)

This is a major aspect of clinical governance and embraces a wide range of issues. Community practitioners need to be aware of what clinical risk structures are in place within their organisation and have access to information associated with these. Clinical risk not only embraces the quality, style, knowledge and skills associated with care. It also needs to consider health and safety and human resource issues as they impact on service delivery.

Moving and handling

Moving and handling is particularly important, as this needs an ongoing training programme within the organisation. The appropriate lifting and moving equipment needs to be purchased to fit the care environment and the needs of the individual. This equip-

---

Box 4.6: Components of clinical risk management

Health and safety
Infection control
Complaints
Incidents reporting
Competence
Policy procedures and protocols
Standards
Information
Knowledge
Record keeping and documentation

---

ment needs to be maintained and updated from time to time. Some district nurses have great difficulty getting the right equipment to the patient as soon as it is required due to organisational and financial constraints. Practitioners have a duty to identify the shortcomings to the organisation (NHS trust) and insist upon the provision of adequate and safe equipment to enable care to be undertaken effectively and safely.

Infection control

The Infection Control Service should also provide updated meaningful advice about microbiological issues and management of infectious patients and equipment (*see* Box 4.7).

Community practitioners should invite the infection control specialist to update them on current thinking around particular aspects of healthcare, such as the management of patients in the community with MRSA, the change in the use of antibiotic therapy in the management of undifferentiated infections, the recent statistical evidence of wound infection rates locally, benchmarked against national trends, or the use of new equipment for the sterilisation of instruments, etc.

Caseload and workload management

Community practitioners need to be reviewing caseloads as these often cause concern related to the pressure practitioners are under to deliver a safe service. Practitioners should be clear that what we are really discussing is *workload*, which is the *active* client/patients

---

Box 4.7: Infection control

When did you and your practice last have a review of your environment to ensure that it was safe with little or no risk of cross infection?

When did you last invite the infection control specialist to update you on their areas of expertise?

---

on the caseload. Workload can vary from day to day, but this must be managed and documented and when pressures of work are continually high and overloading the practitioner.

Community practitioners have a duty to:

• inform management in writing of the difficulties they are experiencing and why

• agree a solution between practitioner and manager

• set a review date, to reassess the situation.

Clinical risk management is partly about managing workload effectively and efficiently, and making professional decisions based on the individual patients' and clients' needs at any one time.

Incidents and complaints

Learning from adverse incidents or complaints is another critical aspect of clinical risk management. An adverse incident may include:

• missed medication at the desired time

• the wrong treatment being administered

• the wrong diagnosis

• inappropriate investigations

• poor assessment techniques.

Complaints often relate to:

- the attitude of the practitioner towards the patient, user or carer
- lack of information
- poor or inappropriate treatment
- poor communication.

It is essential to review practice following an incident or complaint. In many cases necessary actions may include:

- retraining
- redeployment
- environmental changes
- organisational policy changes
- procedure changes.

Clinical audit can be very helpful in monitoring the changes and providing a basis for ongoing learning. Case discussion and peer review using a critical incident technique can also help improve clinical practice following an incident.

Human resources

Many human resource strategies also come under the umbrella of risk management, particularly those associated with:

- violence to staff and patients
- bullying in the work place
- equal opportunities.

These are significant workforce issues and the NHS organisations including PCGs need to have strategies in place to deal with them. Patients can not only use physical violence, but can also verbally abuse staff, which can be damaging and intimidating.

NHS organisations must ensure they have good policies in place that reflect the management of these issues so that staff can obtain support when necessary. Without these supporting mechanisms in place, the NHS trust or organisation could be leaving itself liable to charges of clinical neglect.

Be aware that clinical risk management is about identifying areas at risk and undertaking regular monitoring and review, either by using the audit cycle or benchmarking. Benchmarking is the process of seeking, finding, implementing and sustaining best practice, by comparing the clinical risk policies and strategies with other similar organisations. It prevents 'reinventing the wheel', and enables best practice to become the norm. This methodology can be used both internally within the organisation or externally with other trusts and practices by comparing common aspects. Aspects of clinical risk management should be included as part of an individual's professional development plan, to ensure that they understand the issues associated with risk and how these can be minimised and averted. Some organisations maintain complex policies, procedures and protocols for risk management, but these are only part of the picture. Without the infrastructure to inform, train and educate staff in clinical risk management, policies will not work effectively or efficiently.

Policies, procedures and protocols (PPP)

Clinical governance will demand that organisations have clear policies, procedures and protocols in place, as the chief executive of the NHS trust or chair of the PCG, who is ultimately accountable for clinical governance, will want reassurance that practitioners are practising safely. However, too many restrictive policies do not enable good practice to grow and develop. Those policies, procedures and protocols that are essential should embrace, where appropriate:

• the National Service Framework

• the national guidance that emanates from the National Institute of Clinical Excellence (NICE) (see Box 4.8)

• the local Health Improvement Programme (HImP)

• the evidence, based on research, or high quality evaluated practice.

The community practitioner should:

- enquire locally and nationally about what clinical policies, procedures and protocols are in place or are being developed, before they undertake this task for themselves

- share knowledge, expertise and experience between and across such organisations as social services, PCGs, NHS trusts, health authorities and regions

- involve users and carers in the development or updating of policies, procedures and protocols, as their perspective is extremely valuable

- ensure that all policies are relevant, have a review date and are known to all practitioners

- obtain up-to-date dissemination lists for new policies

- insist on a training programme with the introduction of any new, or updated policies: this is an essential part of the development framework and must be built into the individual's personal development plan

- set time aside to consider PPPs and how they affect practice.

Other aspects of clinical governance that would be part of the community practitioner's work would be the development of professional standards. Many will be unidisciplinary in nature, but as PCGs develop, and partnerships with local health authority colleagues increase, shared standards should be considered, using a methodology that is acceptable to all. In the past, nursing has used the Donabedian methodology, looking at structure, process and outcome. This could be a good place to start the development of shared standards.

Professional accountability

Clinical governance is about professional accountability, not only for your own practice, but also that of others. Working in primary care teams, community practitioners will need to be working in partnership with other key players, including GPs, practice

Box 4.8: The National Institute of Clinical Excellence six-stage approach

Stage 1: Identification
>   for *new* health interventions – 'scanning the horizon' (that is, identifying at an early stage through available intelligence) for new interventions, including drugs, devices and procedures which are likely to have a significant impact on the NHS

>   for existing interventions – examining current practice to identify unjustified variations in use, or uncertainty about clinical and cost-effectiveness

Stage 2: Evidence collection – undertaking research to assess the clinical and cost-effectiveness of health interventions

Stage 3: Appraisal and guidance – carefully considering the implications for clinical practice of the evidence on clinical and cost-effectiveness and producing guidance for the NHS

Stage 4: Dissemination of the guidance and supporting audit methodologies

Stage 5: Implementation at a local level, through clinical governance and other approaches

Stage 6: Monitoring the impact and keeping advice under review, taking into account the views of patients and their representatives and any relevant new research findings

managers and other professional colleagues. If a colleague is not performing to an acceptable standard, then you have a duty to help improve the individual or ensure that help is sought. This duty of care extends throughout the NHS and, where relevant, in the private sector.

Information technology

The September 1998 White Paper *Information for Health* stresses the importance of electronic records. These will be more convenient for patients, and will provide access for all healthcare professionals to the core necessary details, which will be beneficial to the integration of care and can be linked to identifying health outcomes. To implement the framework of clinical governance requires a programme of quality improvement as identified earlier, through clinical audit, evidence-based practice, developing monitoring systems and up-to-date clinical record systems. To achieve this, information can be drawn from:

- local clinical audit data

- national comparative data

- local care pathways

- clinical protocols

- national best practice guidelines from the National Institute of Clinical Excellence

- international research evidence.

Community practitioners will need to develop informatics skills to be able to take advantage of these developments.

Further reading

Community Practitioners' and Health Visitors' Association (October 1998) *Clinical Effectiveness Information Pack*. CPHVA, London.
DoH (1998) *A First Class Service: quality in the new NHS*. The Stationery Office, London.
DoH (1997) *The New NHS: modern, dependable*. HMSO, London.
Health Risk Resource International (June 1998) *Health Risk Resource Pack*. HRRI, London.
Health Visitors' Association (1996) *Quality Counts: an introductory guide to clinical audit in primary care*. HVA, London.
NHS Executive (March 1998) *Achieving Effective Practice: a clinical effectiveness and research information pack for nurses, midwives and health visitors*. NHSE, Leeds.

5

Future developments

Jackie Carnell, Rosemary Cook and Thelma Sackman

The aim of this chapter is to review some of the many different developments in nursing practice and education, as well as in the structure of primary care, which are currently affecting community practitioners, or will do so in the near future. Although the changes brought about by *The New NHS* have taken centre stage, it is important that nurses and health visitors working in primary care see these changes in the wider context, because:

- for all community practitioners, each of these developments has the potential to change the way they work with their patients and clients (more practitioners prescribing, use of video and electronic links to other practitioners during a consultation)

- they change the range and type of services available to clients (additional family support services, choice of telephone or direct 'first contact' service)

- they change the nature of the problems and dependency of patients in primary care (patients requiring comprehensive clinical support nursed at home, people with severe mental illness living in the community)

- for nurses and health visitors on PCG boards, these developments bring together issues of cost, skill mix, workforce planning, service and professional development, and ethics, which have to be resolved into commissioning decisions.

Later in the chapter, these changes and their impact are integrated into a picture of how the community practitioner of the future might work.

Concurrent developments

Table 5.1 shows some of the changes affecting the nursing and health visiting professions, under three headings:

- nursing education
- primary care context
- nursing practice.

Table 5.1 Simultaneous developments affecting nursing

Education	Context	Practice

Specialist practice
Higher level of
  practice
	PCG development
	Ending of internal market
	Health Action Zones
	Recruitment/retention
	  crisis in nursing/
	  general practice
	New family support policies
	IT developments
		Nurse prescribing
		PCAPs pilots
		NHS Direct
		Secondary/primary
		  shift

Now		

Future	Primary care trusts
	IT developments:
	  EPR/EHR
	Increased public
	  involvement
		Outcome of UKCC
		  review
		Roll-out of
		  prescribing
		Telemedicine/telecare
		Strategy for nursing

Nursing education

Specialist practice has been defined by the UKCC as a level of practice attained by registered nurses in which they exercise higher levels of judgement and discretion in clinical care. Specialist practitioner programmes are degree-level educational programmes, lasting one academic year of full-time study, and comprising 50% theory and 50% practice. They cover four areas:

- clinical nursing practice
- care and programme management
- clinical practice development
- clinical practice leadership.

The Specialist Community Practitioner qualification can be obtained in one of eight areas of community nursing:

- general practice nursing
- community mental health nursing
- community learning disability nursing
- community children's nursing
- public health nursing – health visiting
- occupational health nursing
- community nursing in the home – district nursing
- school nursing.

Many existing community practitioners are already specialist practitioners by virtue of their original community qualification, or through programmes undertaken during the 'transitional period' which ended in October 1998. New staff in the community will need to decide whether they wish to pursue a specialist practitioner programme.

A Higher Level of Practice is the title of a UKCC consultation document, published in 1998, which explored the options for recognition of developing nursing practice. It proposed that the UKCC will set a UK-wide, generic standard for a higher level of practice, which is applicable across all healthcare settings. This will be matched by local determination of appropriate knowledge and skill requirements for particular areas of practice. Assessment proposals include:

- the practitioner collecting evidence of their own practice competence in a clinical setting

- confirmation from clinical colleagues and employers of the practitioner's competence

- the production of a written reflective account in a supervised setting

- final assessment at a panel interview.

Prerequisites for assessment are shown in Box 5.1.

Box 5.1: Prerequisites for assessment for higher level of practice

- Current first level registration with the UKCC

- Spend the majority of practice planning and organising, carrying out and evaluating work related to improving health and well being

- Hold a UK degree or equivalent in nursing, midwifery, health visiting or a health related subject, *or*

- Hold a UK degree or equivalent in any other subject together with the successful completion of a post-registration education programme in their area of practice

- Have practised for a specified minimum period of time in their chosen area of practice, probably at least 5000 hours (equivalent to three years full time) in order to collect the required evidence

Primary care context

Primary care group (PCG) formation and the ending of the internal market in healthcare are the focus of the rest of this book. Their significance, and their impact on community nursing both now and in the future, should not be underestimated.

Primary care trusts are the new health service organisations which, it is envisaged, will develop from successful PCGs. They will incorporate the functions and responsibilities of the current community trusts and PCGs, including employing community nurses. Their impact is discussed in detail in Chapter 6.

Public involvement in healthcare has become increasingly important in recent years. There is a lay representative on every PCG board, who helps to ensure that the voice of the service user is contributing to the business of assessing needs and commissioning healthcare for a population. Community practitioners working within the PCG should ensure that they are familiar with the lay representative, who can act as a channel to the board for their own clients' concerns or priorities. Equally, it is important that the lay person on the board has a clear view of the functions, responsibilities and activities of community nurses and health visitors, as they will be involved in commissioning and development decisions affecting their services.

The wider public will also be participating in an annual national survey of patients' and users' experience of the NHS. The survey will consider aspects of care such as access to services, information, technical care, privacy and dignity. Primary and community care were the focus of the first national survey in autumn 1998. Results of the survey will be given to Regional Offices of the NHS Executive, and they will require action plans from health authorities and PCGs to address areas of concern.

The revitalisation of the public health agenda is extremely welcome. The Government Green Paper *Our Healthier Nation* set out a new strategy based on action to address social, economic and environmental factors which lead to poor health and inequalities in health. The goals of *Our Healthier Nation* are shown in Box 5.2. This emphasis on public health will demand a great deal of community practitioners' time, and will become a part of the

---

Box 5.2: *Our Healthier Nation goals*

Aims

- To improve the health of the population as a whole by increasing the length of people's lives and the number of years people spend free from illness

- To improve the health of the worst off in society and to narrow the health gap

Settings for action

- Schools – focusing on children

- Workplaces – focusing on adults

- Neighbourhoods – focusing on older people

Specific targets for 2010

- Heart disease and stroke: to reduce the death rate amongst people under 65 by at least a further third

- Accidents: to reduce accidents by at least a fifth

- Cancer: to reduce the death rate from cancer amongst people under 65 by at least a further fifth

- Mental health: to reduce the death rate from suicide and undetermined injury by at least a further sixth

---

everyday practice of all community nurses. All community practitioners have a major role to play in promoting the health of local communities, through disease prevention and health promotion initiatives. In addition, practitioners on PCG boards, and specialist subgroups or working groups advising the board, will influence primary care commissioning of public health activities.

Health Action Zones (HAZs) are new initiatives which bring together organisations within and beyond the NHS to develop and implement a locally agreed strategy for improving the health of local people. Their emphasis is on partnership and innovation, focusing on areas of deprivation and poor health. Innovative

---

Box 5.3: Statement on family life from *Supporting Families*

'Family life is the foundation on which our communities, our society and our country are built.'

---

projects or service developments can be driven by nurses and health visitors who want to change practice for the benefit of their patients or clients. All community practitioners will need to know whether they are in a designated HAZ area.

Supporting Families is a Government Green Paper issued for consultation in October 1998. It sets out the Government's view about the importance of family life (*see* Box 5.3), and emphasises the important role of the health visitor in embracing the whole well being of parents and children, rather than just their physical

---

Box 5.4: Support for families proposed in *Supporting Families*

- Health visitor input into antenatal classes
- Weekly visits by a health visitor for the first six weeks of a baby's life
- Child health clinics
- Group work giving advice on weaning
- Sleep clinics, helping parents with techniques to establish regular sleeping patterns for their children
- Toddler training groups
- Early relationships groups, dealing with problems such as sibling rivalry
- Advice surgeries, with health visitor availability
- School-setting groups, run jointly by health visitors, school nurses, education staff and GPs, addressing discipline and development of co-operation, prevention of abuse, avoidance of accidents, childhood infections, etc.
- Teenage years groups, helping parents to manage conflict and discipline

---

health. It suggests that health visitors might be required to provide a wide range of support activities, many of which are well established already for some practitioners (*see* Box 5.4). Although the emphasis in the document is on health visitors, midwives are also mentioned for their significant role in the ante- and postnatal period. Other community practitioners also have vital roles to play: school nurses and practice nurses will use their extensive knowledge of local families, as well as their clinical expertise and experience, to provide support in many forms to families.

Sure Start is another support scheme for families. Rather than being universally available, however, it targets geographical areas of greatest need by offering support to parents and children. This support may include:

- training for work
- help with literacy and numeracy
- help and advice on discipline or other parenting problems
- more specific support for the families of children with learning difficulties and emotional and behavioural problems.

Health visitors and other community practitioners will need to identify whether their locality will be a designated Sure Start scheme, as this may offer additional resources to the families with whom they work.

Developments in information technology, and in the way it is used, have been changing the way that nurses work for many years. From the requirement to collect and input statistics for monitoring and contracting purposes, to the receipt of pathology results and updated registration information by direct electronic links to trusts and health authorities, few areas of practice have remained untouched. The recently published NHS information technology strategy makes it clear that further developments are to be given high priority. These include:

- connecting all computerised GP practices to the NHSnet (*see* Box 5.5) by March 2000

- ensuring that GPs and others in primary care can request laboratory tests, receive results, make referrals and book appointments using the NHSnet by March 2002

- introducing electronic patient records (EPRs) in acute hospitals to record treatment and care, and support clinical messaging to primary care

- developing electronic health records (EHRs) in primary care, containing information about patient contacts with the primary healthcare team, as well as summary information about treatment by hospitals and other parts of the NHS. The EHR will be accessible to authorised clinicians, in carefully

---

Box 5.5: The NHSnet

The NHSnet is an 'information superhighway': a secure national network for the delivery of health-related information. Current applications include:

- the NHS Managed Message Handling Service

- the NHS-wide Clearing Service

- access to the Internet

- the NHS Web – a collection of web-based services, currently including an 'NHS Information Zone', where a Directory lists other sites of relevance to the NHS and the delivery of healthcare.

Current NHSnet services include:

- access to computer systems

- videoconferencing

- telemedicine

- distance learning applications

Any GP practice or NHS organisation can connect to the NHSnet, subject to meeting the requirements of the NHSnet Code of Connection: these include the organisation's internal network meeting the baseline requirements of the NHS IM&T Security Policy

---

prescribed circumstances, 24 hours a day

- setting up a national reference library of accredited clinical material on the NHSnet – the National Electronic Library for Health (NELH) – accessible to health professionals through local intranets

- providing access for NHS patients to accredited, independent, multimedia background information and advice about their condition.

Recruitment and retention problems are continuing to affect the nursing profession as a whole, and community nursing is not immune from these problems. The numbers of applications for training places in nursing are falling, while the current nursing population as a whole is ageing. The proportion of nurses under the age of 30 has halved, while those in their 40s and 50s is increasing. One quarter of the total nursing workforce, and 28% of health visitors, will be eligible for retirement in the next five years. General practice is facing a similar phenomenon, with a decline in GP recruitment and a shift towards part-time working with the increase in numbers of female doctors. These issues will need to be addressed if primary care is to achieve its present identified priorities. Retention of current employees needs to be given serious consideration by all NHS employers. Family friendly policies, flexible working conditions, and good terms and conditions of service are essential elements of the solution to the problem of retention. The new human resources strategy for the NHS, *Working Together*, sets out a clear agenda for action on these issues, and will form essential guidance for PCG board members as they seek primary care trust status.

'Skill mix' has been a preoccupation within nursing for some years. In the move towards a workforce that has 'the right skills for the job', community nursing services have introduced staff nurse posts to support district nursing, health visiting and school nursing services. Practice nursing has generally not introduced skill mix to the same degree. PCG boards will have to consider the projected demographic changes in the workforce in primary care, and consider whether they need to change the skills profile and responsibilities of the practitioners in the group

in order to maintain the most effective and safest services to patients.

Nursing practice

Nurse prescribing was piloted in eight GP fundholding practices in 1994, extended to a whole district community trust in 1996, and in 1997 to a further community trust in each region. The national roll-out commenced in the winter of 1998, and will be completed by 2001. This development will mean that all qualified district nurses and health visitors (and practice nurses with a district nursing or health visiting qualification) will be able to prescribe, using the limited Nurse's Formulary (*see* Box 5.6), once they have completed the required training, specified by the English National Board. Community practitioners will want to be involved in discussions about extending the formulary to ensure that it keeps abreast of current practice.

Primary Care Act Pilots (PCAPs) are projects which institute and evaluate different models of primary healthcare service provision. They were set up under the NHS (Primary Care) Act 1997, and around 100 pilots started in April 1998, with more planned for April 1999. The projects range from modest changes in service delivery by GPs, to a small number of nurse-led services in which patients see the nurse as their first contact with primary care services, with, if necessary, referral on to a salaried GP, employed by the nurses through their trust.

NHS Direct is a nurse-led telephone help line for the public, providing advice on health and health services. Nurses are using information technology in the form of computerised 'decision support systems', or protocols, to enable them to advise a caller on:

• what self-help they may require

• whether they need to see a GP

• whether they require urgent hospitalisation.

The decision support software contains detailed algorithms that

Box 5.6: The Nurse Prescribing Formulary

The NPF has 15 sections from which nurses can prescribe:

- laxatives
- analgesics
- local anaesthetics
- drugs for the mouth
- ear wax removal treatments
- drugs for threadworms
- drugs for scabies and head lice
- skin preparations
- disinfection and cleansing
- wound management products
- elastic hosiery
- urinary catheters and appliances
- stoma care products
- appliances and reagent for diabetes
- fertility and gynaecology products

systematically lead the nurse and caller through a series of questions before the final advice is given to the caller. NHS Direct is due to be extended across the country by the year 2001. This service has the potential to influence the way in which primary care is provided in the future, and the way in which the public use their 'first contact' services, such as GPs and community nurses.

Developments in information technology, as well as changing the way in which information is handled and shared between health professionals and across organisational boundaries, will also change the way clinical care is given. Telemedicine services already exist, allowing specialists at a distance from the patient to give an opinion on their condition through the use of video and telecommunications links. Existing examples include:

- the transmission of fetal monitoring data from women at home via telephone lines to midwives in other locations

- consultations between GPs and specialists on dermatological conditions, using video and computer technology.

Similar developments also allow nurse practitioners to have instant access to GPs on different sites, for live consultation about patients who need a medical opinion.

As PCGs begin to act as organisations, rather than individual practices, they may consider the benefits of sharing skilled personnel between practices, or creating peripatetic posts. The ability to transmit and consult on clinical data, between nurse and doctor or between nurse and nurse, in 'real time', will contribute enormously to both clinical safety and the convenience of the service to the patient.

The shift from secondary to primary care, which has been gathering pace in recent years, will continue to change the dependency of patients nursed in primary care, and so require new skills and ways of working from community practitioners. This shift has already led to developments such as:

- rapid response teams, which move in quickly to provide the support and care necessary to prevent an admission to hospital, for both physical and mental illness

- 'intermediate care teams', which provide intensive levels of multi-disciplinary support, to allow people to be discharged home from hospital much earlier than usual

- clinical nurse specialists in conditions such as diabetes, for example, who work principally in primary care, allowing diabetic patients to be stabilised on insulin without admission to hospital

- community children's nursing teams, which allow children with serious or life-limiting conditions to be given specialised, comprehensive nursing care at home, minimising or removing the need for admissions to secondary care.

Community practitioners are likely to be already involved with clients living at home who would once have received secondary care. Nurses and health visitors on PCG boards will be considering the costs and benefits of providing services in this way to their population, including assessing the impact on the skill mix and cost of the nursing workforce in the PCG.

Other changes and developments affecting the whole profession, in primary care and elsewhere, include the current review of the Nurses, Midwives and Health Visitors Act, which may change the system of registering and recording professional qualifications, and the imminent publication of the new strategy for nursing. The development of the profession as a whole, as well as changes to the everyday practice of individual nurses, health visitors and midwives, takes place in the context of the structural changes to the health service and developments in education described here.

A view of the future

Although there are four different agendas across the United Kingdom, the desires underpinning all of them are:

• to modernise the NHS

• to develop radically different ways of delivering services.

The most important ingredient in this radical approach to delivering services is the development of close working partnerships between:

• all NHS professionals

• other agencies

• the general public.

An example of this drive towards working in partnership is being given to us by this Government, developing policies which have implications for, and have been developed by, a range of Government departments. The Department of Health, the Home Office, the Treasury and the Department for Education and Employment, for example, have developed the emerging family policies. The main aim of the public health Green Paper *Our Healthier Nation* is to tackle social exclusion and reduce the inequality gap. Within these agendas for the health services, what does the future hold for community practitioners and health visitors?

Firstly, this future has to be viewed in context, not just of the NHS agendas, but in the broader context in which the NHS operates. There is emerging consensus that we are at the threshold of a new sociotechnological age. This age will be the product of emerging technology, which will bring with it open access for the general public to knowledge and information formerly only available to professionals, as well as technological advancements which will mean that some present occupations will disappear. An example of the former is the NHS Web, which will have on it information about conditions and the best practice in their treatment, with supporting evidence. Ninety per cent of this Web will be open to the public. An example of the latter is shown in Box 5.7.

Speaking at the Chief Nursing Officer's Conference in November 1998, Sir Alan Langlands, Chief Executive of the NHS Executive, gave six predictions for the new millennium:

- the pace of the therapeutic revolution will increase

- the pace of the IT revolution will increase

- the impact of changes in our physical environment will be felt, including global warming, changes in the pattern of communicable diseases and the effects of genetically engineered crops

- there will be less tolerance of shortcomings in the NHS

- there will be increasing 'globalisation'

- there will be a move away from hierarchical working: the new currencies will be knowledge, skill, innovation and autonomy.

Discussing the kind of leaders needed for this new world, Professor Jean Faugier suggested that they will need to:

- determine the forward direction

- remove the obstacles

> **Box 5.7:** An example of technological advancement in healthcare
>
> Dr Tim Porter O'Grady, speaking at the Chief Nursing Officer's conference in 1998, described how he had been nearly blind and needed strong glasses, with many trips to his local optometrist. Laser technology brought him 20/20 vision in 7½ minutes.

- develop ownership

- stimulate self-directed action.

A manager from British Telecom listed the drivers which are increasing the use of information technology, in healthcare as elsewhere:

- labour-related costs are increasingly expensive

- there is an expertise and skill shortage

- IT has the ability to enhance communications

- IT and communications are decreasing in price.

The challenges for the future are:
- to give everyone basic IT literacy

- to empower the users of IT

- to create an open, sharing culture

- to manage anarchy.

The role of community practitioners

The role of health visitors and community practitioners will be crucial to delivering the new NHS agenda, but they have to be allowed to do so. They are the professionals, who, with their GP colleagues, best understand the individuals, families and communities they serve. They can forge powerful local partnerships with all the relevant parties to drive local Health Improvement

Programmes forward. They are best placed to focus the attentions and commitment of others on action to address social exclusion and reduce local health inequalities. However, to drive effective and radically different services, they in turn have to be commissioned in effective and radically different ways. Commissioning currency has to be expressed in terms of outcomes, not inputs. And, since quantifying outcomes is inherently more challenging than quantifying inputs, risk management is a skill that has to be acquired by all concerned (*see* Box 5.8). All community practitioners and health visitors now have to be called to account for what they achieve, not what they do. There has to be shared understanding of what the desired outcomes are. Those who work in the community should determine how these outcomes should be achieved within a community setting. Authority has to be given to those doing the job to prescribe their own practice, forge their own partnerships and evaluate results. They can then be called to account for their practice against what is known to be clinically effective, research-based practice, and what they are achieving against agreed outcomes. Process measures have to be accepted when real health gains, for individual, families and communities, might not be determined for five, ten or even 15 years.

This workforce will need leaders who reflect the attributes already listed. Management by command and control, appropriate for the industrial age, must now make way for leaders who create the environment in which equitable partnerships can be developed to deliver creative and relevant services to individuals, families and communities. Community practitioners and health visitors have to acquire these leadership skills necessary for the new age themselves, as well as providing inspirational leadership to the multi-skilled team they will be leading.

Box 5.8: The need to learn to manage risk

Speaking to nurse leaders about the changing context for nursing and healthcare, Dr Tim Porter O'Grady said:

'If you define new outcomes, and do not change practice, insanity follows.'

The workforce of the future has to be more flexible. There will be no room for any group of professionals who cannot articulate and demonstrate their contribution to the overall outcomes for the future. In an NHS where technological advances, and advances in knowledge, might make one group redundant, re-skilling and re-education for new roles must become acceptable and exciting rather than unacceptable and frightening. The NHS of the future cannot afford to consign any of its workforce to the scrapheap.

Within this new age and new NHS, the future for community practitioners is as bright as they wish to make it. One obvious fact that could mitigate against this is the decline in the number of people entering the nursing profession as a whole. The numbers of people entering health visiting and district nursing training had fallen by just over 50% from 1990 to 1996, but is now rising marginally. Extra investment in those entering specialist community practice is essential: they are our leaders of tomorrow.

In *Perceptions of Nursing as a Career*, a report for the Department of Health, it was reported that young people's perceptions were:

- that caring is the role of a subordinate

- that helping is a leadership role and seen as synonymous with medicine

- that caring attributes are seen as female

- that girls will consider 'male', high status work but boys will not consider 'female work' which is seen as low status

- that young people admire those who choose to enter nursing, but do not envy them or desire to enter nursing themselves.

It is suggested in the report that nursing and its status would be enhanced by the establishment of a common basis for medical training in higher education, shared between nursing, medicine and professions allied to medicine. As well as helping to recruit nurses, this might also lay firm foundations for positive partnerships between NHS professionals. However, it would be necessary to ensure that the training and education of nurses equipped them with a broad range of skills, and a robust attitude to change, which includes the acceptance that re-skilling for new roles is likely to be necessary at least once in a career. Education itself has to be provided in a flexible format, with all professional education being seen as relevant and transferable.

The future NHS, in the context of the evolving new age, will provide a stimulating and challenging environment for community practitioners and health visitors to work in. A new age will call for a more assertive and confident nursing profession that can adapt and change to a climate of evolving need.

Further reading

DoH (1998) *Supporting Families: a consultation document*. The Stationery Office, London.

NHS Executive (1998) *Information for Health: an information strategy for the modern NHS, 1998–2005*. NHSE, Leeds.

UKCC (1998) *A Higher Level of Practice: a consultation document*. UKCC, London.

6

Primary care trusts

Rosemary Cook

The aim of this chapter is to describe the structure proposed for primary care trusts (PCTs), and the way they will operate. It will also highlight the differences between primary care groups (PCGs) and PCTs, and discuss the implications of PCTs for community practitioners.

PCTs: first signs

Primary care trusts, like primary care groups, were first described in the White Paper, *The New NHS: modern, dependable*. They were the 'freestanding options' of Level 3 and Level 4 PCGs (*see* Box 6.1). Such trusts could only be established by new legislation, and the focus of the White Paper was largely on the Level 1 and Level 2 PCGs, which would be forerunners of primary care trusts. However, some key characteristics of PCTs were outlined in the White Paper:

- they would be managed by a Board of GPs, community nurses and managers

- they would hold a unified budget of General Medical Services

---

Box 6.1: The four levels of PCGs

Level 1 – acts in an advisory capacity to the health authority
Level 2 – takes devolved responsibility for managing the budget for healthcare in the area, acting as part (a sub-committee) of the health authority
Level 3* – a freestanding body accountable to the health authority for commissioning care
Level 4* – a freestanding body accountable to the health authority for commissioning care, and with added responsibility for providing community services for their population

*These are PCTs requiring new legislation (contained in the Health Bill currently before Parliament)

---

cash-limited allocations, hospital and community health services funding, and prescribing allocations

- they would employ all relevant community health staff and run community hospitals and other community facilities

- they would not be expected to take responsibility for specialised mental health or learning disability services.

The White Paper also spelt out some criteria for PCGs to move to independent PCT status (*see* Box 6.2).

Box 6.2: Criteria for the move from PCG to PCT status

- Proper arrangements for financial accountability

- Well-developed arrangements for monitoring activity and developing practice-led clinical standards

- Making an effective contribution and working within the HImP set by the health authority and partner organisations

- Agree standards and targets set with the health authority

- Broad support locally for the establishment of such a trust

PCTs: 'establishing better services'

A Department of Health document, *Primary Care Trusts: establishing better services*, published in April 1999, sets out much more detailed guidance on the formation and structure of PCTs.

PCTs will be free-standing, statutory bodies, responsible for delivering better health and better care to their local population. The legislation required to set up such bodies is contained within the Health Bill, currently receiving its second reading in Parliament. PCTs will operate at one of two levels:

- Level 3 trusts will commission services and employ a limited range of staff

- Level 4 trusts will be able to provide community health services as well as commission other health services, run community hospitals, employ the necessary staff, and own property.

The precise range of services provided will vary according to local circumstances, and will be decided on during the local consultation process which precedes the setting up of the trust (*see* below). The local health authority will delegate to the PCT responsibility for securing the necessary health services for the local population, and the PCT will be accountable to the health authority for delivering them. Some of the functions to be retained by the health authority are shown in Box 6.3.

All primary care trusts will have three overall functions which

---

Box 6.3: Functions to be retained by the health authority

- Strategic planning
- Regulatory functions
- Commissioning of very specialist services
- Responsibility for dental, optical and pharmacy services
- Payment of GPs' fees and allowances
- Disciplinary functions

mirror those of the PCGs from which they have developed:

- to improve the health of the local community
- to develop primary and community health services
- to commission secondary care services.

PCTs will not be able to provide general medical services which will continue to be provided by GPs working as independent contractors.

PCT partnerships and links

PCTs will have to work in partnership with NHS trusts, hospital doctors and local medical, optical and pharmaceutical committees. They will also need to develop links with community health councils and local voluntary groups.

Governing the PCTs

Both Level 3 and Level 4 PCTs will have a Board, typically consisting of 11 members. These will be:

- a Chair, appointed by the Secretary of State (as in current NHS trusts)
- five lay members, appointed by the Secretary of State (as in current trusts)
- a Chief Executive
- a Finance Director
- three professional members: usually a Clinical Governance Director, a nurse and a GP.

The Chair and Board will be accountable to the local health authority and, ultimately, to the Secretary of State.

As well as a Board, each trust will have an Executive which deals with day-to-day decision making and strategic development.

The Board and the Executive will work closely together in order to run the trust. However, the Board will retain sole responsibility for some key decisions (*see* Box 6.4). The composition of the Executive differs between Level 3 and Level 4 trusts. In Level 3 trusts, it mirrors the Board of Level 1 and 2 PCGs, with the addition of a public health or health promotion professional. Level 4 trusts will have ten clinicians on the Executive 'with significant representation from general practice balanced with local nurses and community and public health professionals.' Figure 6.1 shows the full composition of the Boards and Executives of Level 3 and 4 trusts.

Box 6.4: Decisions to be made solely by the PCT Board

- Remuneration of Executive members
- Proposals for expenditure on GMS infrastructure
- Establishing GMS local development schemes
- Entering into contracts for services under the Primary Care Act.

Trusts and clinical governance

Like all other NHS bodies and professionals, PCTs will be responsible for clinical governance. In trusts this will mean having:

- clear lines of responsibility and accountability for the overall quality of clinical care (note that the Clinical Governance Director sits on both the Board and the Executive)
- a programme of quality improvements
- education and training plans for staff
- integrated procedures for all professionals to identify and remedy poor professional performance
- clear risk management policies.

Level 3

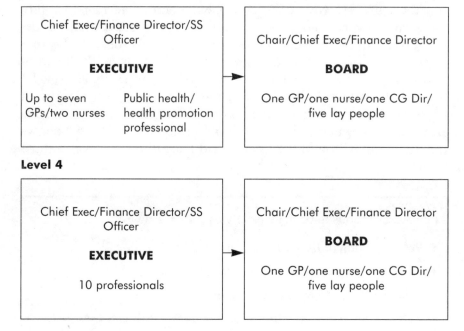

Note: Other alternative governance arrangements may be proposed to suit local needs, and will be considered.

Figure 6.1 Composition of Boards and Executives of PCTs.

PCGs and PCTs compared

Although PCTs will develop from Level 1 and 2 PCGs, there are significant differences between the two forms of local commissioning organisation which have implications for community practitioners. The principal differences are shown in Box 6.5.

How PCTs will begin

Establishing Better Services describes the process by which a Level 2 PCG can progress to become either a Level 3 or 4 primary care trust. The key points are:

Box 6.5: Differences between PCGs and PCTs

PCGs	Trusts
• Are part of the health authority	• Are freestanding, statutory bodies
• Cannot employ staff	• Will employ commissioning (Level 3) and providing (Level 4) staff
• Have a Board but no Executive	• Have a Board and an Executive
• Have a public health or health promotion professional on the Board	• Have 10 places on the Executive for professionals, including public health and social services expertise
• Plan, commission, monitor and develop health services	• Also provide community health services
• Already exist	• Can only be established by the Secretary of State after consultation with local stake-holders

---

- PCTs can only be established by the Secretary of State

- any individual within a PCG, community trust or health authority can generate a proposal to establish a PCT (but the consultation process will only be implemented if the proposal has been endorsed by either the PCG or the community trust)

- the health authority must then co-ordinate a local consultation process on the proposal, involving local PCGs, GPs, other professions, the health and local authorities, NHS trusts and the wider community

- the Secretary of State, acting through the relevant Regional Office, will consider proposals and decide which can be approved.

The first PCTs should be in place by April 2000, with 1999–2000 acting as a development period for them.

PCT staff

Level 3 PCTs will employ only the staff they need for their commissioning role. Level 4 trusts will also employ the staff needed for the provision of community health services and, where this is included in their proposal, the running of community hospitals.

Many of these staff will already be employed within the PCG, community trust or health authority. The Secretary of State will be able to make an order providing for the transfer of these staff to employment by the PCT under the same safeguards as staff transferring under TUPE (the Transfer of Undertakings (Protection of Employment) Regulations 1981). This will mean that staff:

- retain existing terms and conditions of service

- have no break in service

- will continue to be eligible for the NHS pension scheme.

Staff will be consulted before any such transfer order is made. An important point about this transfer is that staff currently working for community trusts will not become employees of GPs or practices. They will transfer from the community trust to the PCT.

PCTs, staff and *Working Together*

In general, new primary care trusts will be expected to demonstrate commitment to the provisions of *Working Together*, the national NHS human resources (HR) framework. MSF has suggested some essential criteria which should be met by PCGs before they become PCTs:

- they must be large enough to meet risk management criteria, including providing skilled and competent general management, HR management, professional leadership and clinical governance

- they must be able to demonstrate how services which may not easily fit into PCTs will be maintained, e.g. midwifery, school nursing, speech and language therapy

- they must be able to demonstrate how their development will be informed by good change management processes and be able to win and maintain the support of all affected groups of staff

- they must demonstrate that they will have the HR capacity, staff numbers, and skills to meet the HR criteria

- they must be committed to the *Positively Diverse* and HR strategy goals of zero tolerance for racism, and improvement in the racial composition of the workforce

- they must be able to demonstrate an understanding of, and commitment to, the full range of grievance procedures and fair disciplinary providers at the standards expected by statute, case law and good HR practice

- they must be able to demonstrate an understanding of, and commitment to, a Health Improvement Programme for all staff

- they must be committed to maximising the opportunities for employing salaried GPs

- they must be committed to openness and transparency in all matters regarding the governance and operations of the PCT, including an understanding of the need to have a whistleblowing procedure

- they must be able to demonstrate an understanding of how to address inter professional conflict in such a way as to meet good standards of HR and professional accountability

- Level 3 PCGs must be able to demonstrate an understanding of the HR implications of the commissioning role, and a willingness and ability to ensure that statutory good practice and NHS national standards will be observed in considering the impact of Level 3 commissioning on staff employed by other NHS organisations

- they must understand the need to have in place clear procedures to ensure that independent contractor GPs will be bound by the above policies and goals.

Implications for community practitioners

For community practitioners currently employed by NHS trusts, the setting up of a Level 4 PCT in their area will mean:

- they will be consulted about the transfer of their employment to the new trust

- they will become employees of the PCT, on the same or better terms and conditions as their current employment, and with continuity of employment and pension rights

- they will be working for an NHS organisation which has a professionally-led executive, and a nurse on the Board.

The opportunities which are beginning to become apparent in PCGs, for community practitioners to contribute to working groups and project teams which advise the Board, will continue. They can also be co-opted onto the Executive, where their expertise can inform day-to-day decisions and the implementation of policy.

Summary

Primary care trusts are the independent, freestanding bodies into which primary care groups are expected to evolve. The Secretary of State will establish PCTs, if appropriate, following full consultation with local stakeholders. Level 3 trusts fulfil commissioning functions, and will only employ staff for this purpose. Level 4 trusts will also provide community health services and employ a range of community staff. These staff will mostly be transferred from current health authority, community trust or PCG employment, with full protection of their employment conditions and rights. MSF has proposed a set of criteria which should be met by PCGs aspiring to become PCTs, to ensure that the national strategic framework for HR in the NHS can be implemented in the new bodies. Community practitioners will have additional opportunities to contribute their essential skills and knowledge through work on, or with, the trust Executive, and through project teams and working groups.

Appendix

An alternative look at the future: PCGs and PCTs
A constellation of interests[*]

Patricia Oakley and Annette Keen

The previous chapters described the recent changes being implemented in the NHS and their implications for nurses and health
visitors who work in the community. This chapter draws on their
insights and looks to the future by assessing how community
nurses and health visitors might be developed under the auspices
of the proposed Health Bill which should become law in 1999. This
appendix therefore examines:

- the current position and the proposals for developing PCGs and
  trusts

- the likely transition agenda and the need to create a more
  consistent, transparent and accountable approach

- the likely management issues in developing new ways of
  working in the future.

The current position and proposals for developing PCGs and trusts

The NHS reforms of 1989 introduced the concept of the 'internal market', separating purchasers from providers of services. This led to the now familiar organisational structures of acute, community and mental health trusts and to the development of GP purchasing groups in the form of fundholders, multi-funds, total purchasing funds and co-operatives. Although introducing the market concept in the NHS was fundamentally flawed, one of the positive lessons of the changes was that clinicians and professional staff, and managers, learnt how to make sense of, and implement, major and difficult organisational changes.

In the subsequent reorganisations, the management structures were streamlined, e.g. the Health Authorities Act of 1995 saw the 14 regional health authorities reduced to eight, and the 90 district health authorities and family health service authorities replaced by new health authorities. While the former regional health authorities were developed into regional offices and emanations of civil service, the new health authorities were empowered to act as the publicly accountable bodies, i.e. statutory authorities, with the authority to spend and account for public money. Currently, they discharge this responsibility through a system of planning and fund allocations and, in some cases, they are able to join with local authorities to jointly plan and purchase specialist services. Despite an easing in the regulations about public finances, health authorities are constrained in their ability to pool budgets and move monies around the system with ease. Therefore, in the main, at the moment, purchasing care from social services, trusts and from GPs remains discrete and poorly integrated.

However, the proposed reforms outlined in the White Paper, *The New NHS: modern, dependable*, will fundamentally change the role of the health authority with the introduction of PCGs, and eventually primary care trusts (PCTs). Subject to the legislative changes, PCGs will be involved in commissioning services and, eventually, PCTs will manage proposed cash allocations for acute and community services within their localities from a single unified health budget.

Nurses and health visitors working in the community should be fully aware of these changes and the impact of this transfer of responsibility on their future management, development and accountability arrangements. The health authority therefore has a critical role in shaping the future development of PCGs and PCTs and, hence, the future of nursing and health visiting practices. The health authority requires support as it has a heavy agenda over the coming years. For instance, it will have to:

- *Keep things going by*:
  - meeting the standing financial instructions (SFIs) and maintaining balanced budgets
  - supporting financial changes which accompany implementation of PCGs
  - managing trust mergers and service reconfigurations
  - managing the proposed changes to the contract currencies
  - implementing the new IM&T Strategy and ensuring year 2000 compliance

- *Establish PCGs (and eventually PCTs) by*:
  - setting up the infrastructures to support PCGs, including the know-how for commissioning and contracts management
  - setting up the structures and processes for establishing good governance procedures, financial and clinical
  - setting up policies and practices for managing staff in accordance with standard good practices
  - delegating, in time, powers of attorney to PCTs
  - coping with the loss of experienced staff who will be attracted to the new posts within PCGs

- *Develop new ways of working with local authorities and, eventually, with the new regional government structures by*:
  - developing closer working partnerships with social services
  - developing links with local education, transport and housing policy development groups as seen in some of the pilot Health and Education Action Zones
  - developing links with local voluntary and community groups
  - getting ready for regional government

– developing new cultures and ways of working.

Given the scope of this agenda and its impact on the people employed in health authorities, nurses and health visitors working in the community and in primary care will need to be sensitive to the fact that implementing these changes will give rise to human complexities, as well as logistical and management problems.

Nevertheless, the likely benefits of empowering PCGs, and eventually PCTs, in this way are evident when we consider their proposed responsibility for determining and delivering strategies for improving the health of local people. The importance of local commissioning groups in planning and in allocating funds for meeting the local needs of patient care cannot be overstated. In developing local agendas for advancing community-based nursing and health visiting practices, individuals will need a thorough understanding of the proposed reforms and their implications.

Following *The New NHS: modern, dependable* PCGs were established as subcommittees of the health authority. It is envisaged that PCGs will act as the fulcrum of change as they mature and develop the necessary infrastructures and know-how to take on the development of local commissioning plans for healthcare; allocating and reconciling budgets against these plans; and developing the necessary structures and processes for public accountability, probity and good governance – both clinical and financial. The health authority's role, acting as the midwife, encompasses the need to develop and support the PCGs so that they become, where appropriate, free-standing legally established PCTs.

The proposals for PCTs include their ability to use the new operational flexibilities to allow them to work more closely with local authorities, to design their own incentive arrangements, and to provide personal medical and dental services under the Primary Care Act, or to enter into local contracts to do so.

On the one hand, this could look like an existing community trust which has developed a closely integrated service with local GPs, through say the locality teams, which starts to employ GPs. On the other hand, it could look like a former multi-fund or co-operative of GPs, organised as a PCG, which takes over the management of the community nursing and health visiting services. The guidance proposes a template but this is flexible, being open to local formulations providing they satisfy four criteria:

1 put primary care professionals in the driving seat

2 provide public accountability

3 support public involvement, with trusts rooted firmly in the local community

4 ensure probity, with robust safeguards both to protect public funds and primary care professionals from suggestions of any conflicts of interest.

Crucially, they must 'avoid being cumbersome or unwieldy' so, within this framework, PCGs, as embryonic PCTs, have to establish their governance structures and management processes, and agendas to deliver these four criteria. At the same time, this new and developing organisational form has to support the implementation of the three interrelated major operational agendas for the service: the clinical governance agenda; the national human resource management strategy; and the information management and technology strategy which includes the prescribing support tool, PRODIGY, and the National Electronic Library for Health, NELH.

Clearly, the workload will be great and it will require very skilled individuals working within the PCGs, and PCTs, to deliver these complex changes while keeping the everyday services going at the normal rate. To tease out the impact for community-based nurses and health visitors, we need to examine the likely details of these proposals and how they fit together in a coherent transitional development phase.

The likely transition agenda

The likely transition agenda will include a start-up phase where local staff begin to make sense of what the proposals might mean in their local contexts; a building phase where the supporting infrastructures are set up and developed to address, in particular, the governance structures and processes to achieve probity and public accountability; and the synergistic parallel building phase where people's skills and knowledge are developed to the level expected of a management team which is going to run a trust with a working budget in the region of £50–60m per year.

The start-up phase

The PCGs will need to set up their infrastructures to develop local health strategies, the macro commissioning agenda and, at the same time, the mechanisms for their translation into managing care delivery with the local care management teams – the micro commissioning agenda.

To do this, PCGs need to set up and develop policy formulation groups constituted around either care groups and/or disease groups. These are likely to include medical, nursing and social care components and an underpinning component of specialist advice on, for instance, prescribing and medicines management, rehabilitation therapy services and any other specialist advice from a respected body.

To formulate their health commissioning policies, PCGs, in their start-up phase, must set up at least three buttressing information systems: from public health, research and other august bodies including the new National Institute for Clinical Excellence (NICE); from the medicines management centre, drug information networks, Medicines Control Agency (MCA) and the Prescription Pricing Bureau (PPB); and from the contracting, activity and financial planning networks. This is summarised in the left-hand side of Figure 1.

Having developed the macro commissioning agenda, PCGs will then have to translate these high level plans into contract currency which allows local practices and care management teams to understand what they are supposed to be doing by way of activity (numbers and care plans) and budgets (the cash allocations for the agreed activities and care plans). In effect, as shown on the right-hand side of Figure 1, the primary and community care teams, operating in a care management system, become accountable to the PCG for their work and may create, in time, a further micro

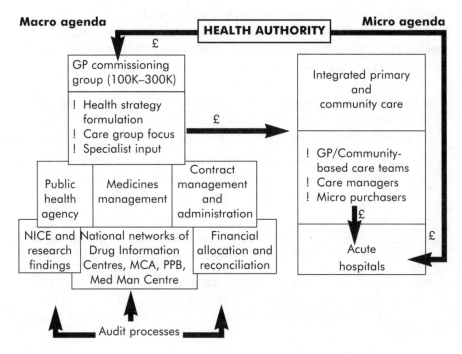

Figure 1 Developing a macro and micro commissioning framework.

commissioning system whereby the community-based care manager 'purchases' secondary care interventions from the local acute hospital provider where necessary.

This might appear at first sight to be rather daunting, but it is, in effect, not dissimilar to the social services care management system already in operation, and many of the foundation stones for such a scheme have already been laid by some of the GP fund-holders and multi-funds. When a similar system was introduced in the USA in the mid-80s, it created tremendous pressure on the acute sector because nurse care managers, operating a community-based care system, did precisely that – they maintained their patients in the community which resulted in a collapse in the cash flows to the local hospitals. Learning from this experience, to prevent any catastrophic failure in the acute sector in the UK context, the health authority would have to manage the cash flows and changes carefully through planned rationalisations. Hence the likely cash flows indicated in Figure 1. Because public money is at stake, the whole system must be subject to audit.

The implications of all this for community-based nurses and health visitors is that specialist practitioners will be needed in time for the following emerging roles:

- commissioning specialists in care and/or disease groups who can access, use and synthesise complex technical data with ease and make sense of these to develop locally coherent health plans

- contracting specialists who can translate these high level plans into a local contract currency which gives local providers the details of the relevant planned activities and finances

- value for money assessors who can assess the quality of the work delivered against the national standards set by NICE and against the budget allocated for the work

- nurse and health visitor care managers who are able to manage a team of qualified support staff and organise their work on a day-to-day basis, and the budgets to go with the contracted activities

- research specialists who are able to work in and with research teams on locally commissioned research programmes using both qualitative and quantitative methodologies and longitudinal research designs.

The building phase for establishing governance structures and processes

As subcommittees of the health authority, and eventually as publicly accountable PCTs, PCGs will need to work on their governance and accountability structure. A possible outline example is shown in Figure 2.

The purpose of the finance and clinical subcommittees is to provide the necessary transparent and accountable structures and processes to show how the finance and clinical quality governance agendas are developed and monitored.

The Standing Policy Steering Groups and their Policy Working Groups form the structure of accountability for the macro commissioning development discussed above. The Standing Committees

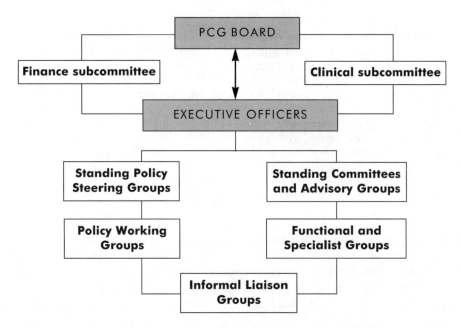

Figure 2 An example of a governance and accountability structure.

and Advisory Groups form the specialist supportive networks which help the Steering and Policy Working Groups to formulate their plans. It is likely, based on current experiences, that functional and specialist groups will inform these advisory bodies. For example, the Maternity Services Liaison Committee, the Therapists' Advisory Councils, and the Pharmacists and Therapeutics Information Advisory Groups already provide such support in many places. Underneath this structure of accountability, the policy decision-making forums might be represented as shown in Figure 3.

The implication of this is that tensions and conflict will more than likely arise naturally and these will need to be resolved by experienced staff trained in brokerage and arbitration techniques. Many nurses and health visitors have natural skills in this area, and have practised such techniques, probably unknowingly, over many years. PCGs might usefully recognise this skill and nurture and develop the individuals who possess it, creating an indigenous brokering and arbitration service.

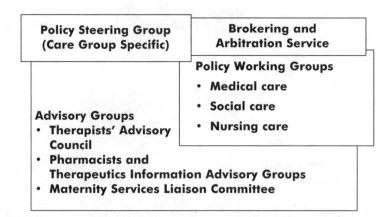

Figure 3 A structure for decision-making and advisory groups.

PCGs will also have to develop their detailed governance structures for financial and clinical quality management. Essentially, this is about setting up and developing the right information flows as shown in Figures 4 and 5, and understanding what the information means.

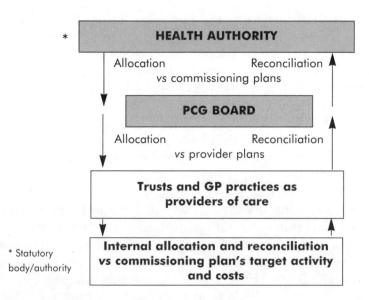

Figure 4 Financial allocation and reconciliation flows.

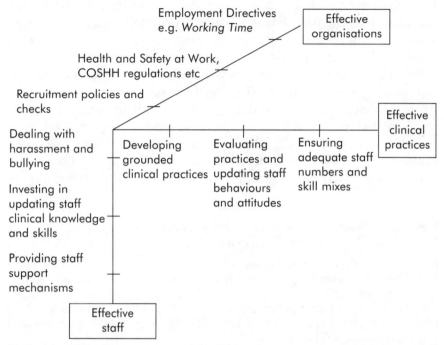

Figure 5 Clinical governance and the human resource management accountability framework.

The implication of these complex and detailed management agendas is that good quality middle and senior managers, who are likely to have clinical backgrounds, will be required to develop the PCG staff's capability to handle the financial and clinical quality issues, including the human resource management issues.

The building phase for establishing skills and knowledge

In time, the current patterns of working need to be changed and the problems with team working resolved through development of a systematic investment programme in people's skills and knowledge. This is likely to be brought into sharp focus as the requirements for continuing practice development and lifelong learning become clearer under the proposed revisions to the Nurses, Midwives and Health Visitors Act, and the likely compulsory reaccreditation for doctors every five years. The RCN has recently published a comprehensive list of skills requirements as shown in Box 1.[1]

Given the heavy pressures on staff time, it is unlikely that the traditional training mechanisms will be suitable as, for example, it will be very difficult for staff to be released for long courses, e.g. up to and over five days. As an alternative, team-based learning mechanisms in situ will need to be developed, supported by individual learning contracts which respect the individual's preferred style. Clearly, this will need resources to support both staff replacement costs and learning costs which include tutors, super-

---

Box 1: The knowledge and skills that primary care nurses need to develop to make PCG/Ts a success

- Current and continued clinical credibility
- Ability to promote good health behaviour and act as an advocate for health
- Knowledge of best practice and the National Service Frameworks ensuring local application of these through a partnership approach
- Audit and quality monitoring
- Research and development skills
- Risk management skills
- Knowledge of the public health approach to healthcare and the ability to generate a health profile of the local population
- Data collection and analysis
- Numeracy skills
- IT skills
- Presentation skills
- Budget and resource management
- Problem-solving skills
- Ability to lead and contribute effectively to nursing and cross-functional teams
- Networking with nurses, health and social care professionals, voluntary agencies and users
- Negotiation, influencing and political sensitivity skills
- Knowledge of the role of the health authority
- Understanding the contribution of primary, secondary and tertiary care and the consortia in meeting the national and local healthcare agenda
- Knowledge of the national and local healthcare agenda and ability to translate this into practice

visors, co-counsellors, access to the internet and journals etc. PCGs will therefore need to think carefully about investment planning in staff and their development needs.

Having invested in their staff PCGs need to retain them by developing, over time, a coherent human resource management policy framework, and operational procedures to deliver the policy's objectives. This should embrace the recruitment and retention of staff, their development and performance appraisal, and ensure that staff are working in a safe environment, both physically and psychologically. Recent case law helps to inform what might be seen as a reasonable minimum starting point. While PCGs are subcommittees of the health authority, recognition of trade unions is not an issue as staff have this right within the current arrangements in community trusts. However, as PCTs develop and employ staff directly, recognition will be a management issue.

Many community-based nurses and health visitors have good experience in managing staff and developing in-service training and audit schemes, and developing robust human resource management practices. PCGs might usefully tap this body of knowledge and experience as they develop and mature their infrastructures, in readiness to become a PCT. A necessary condition of becoming a PCT is likely to be for an organisation to demonstrate that the infrastructures and architecture for accountability and staff management, as discussed before, are in place.

The likely management issues in developing new ways of working in the future

The need for strong leadership and a supportive culture

To develop an understanding of how important PCG/Ts will be in creating a culture which supports a unified approach, it is useful to use Hampden-Turner's model in which he describes the function of culture as 'to try and mediate dilemmas'.[2] Within PCG/Ts there will be daily issues creating dilemmas that express themselves as tensions. If the PCG/T fails to reconcile these dilemmas and tensions, the culture will be unreconciled and even adversarial. Hampden-Turner describes this as a vicious circle because each side of the dilemma:*

'frustrates the other, contends with it and contradicts it'.

The vicious circle does not support efficient or effective growth of the organisation in realising its goals. Indeed, it may never realise its goals and certainly not without expending a great deal more time, energy and resources than it might otherwise do if there was less conflict.

In contrast, if the PCG/T reconciles dilemmas and creates synergy there will be creative tension and mutual restraint and the culture will become self-correcting. Hampden-Turner describes this as a virtuous circle. The harmony and creative tension of a virtuous circle supports the growth of an efficient and effective organisation which realises its goals.

Leadership has a vital role to play in creating a virtuous circle. The key skill in moving these organisations forward arises from the ability of leaders to offer individuals in the organisation a sense of both the dilemmas facing the organisation, and how they can be resolved and reconciled. Within the PCG/T every nurse and health visitor can enhance their individual leadership skills through the acquisition and application of conflict management and negotiation skills in particular, and these skills will help to reconcile the dilemmas facing the PCG/T as a whole. The leadership agenda to reconcile the dilemmas facing PCG/Ts is summarised in Figure 6.

The need for establishing trust as the principal controlling mechanism

The NHS is currently composed of many diverse organisations which have mutual interdependence. To create a more unified approach, a way of working needs to be established that will ensure these individual entities begin to act as a more coherent organisation in the form of a PCT. Birnbirg describes four points on a continuum of involvement between such organisations, as illustrated in Figure 7. [3]

* In Greek *dilemma* means literally 'two propositions'.

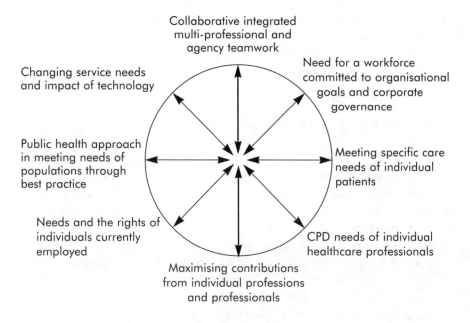

Figure 6 The leadership agenda to reconcile the dilemmas facing PCGs/PCTs.

At present, the relationship between most NHS organisations in this continuum might be described as customer supplier, or sole source supplier, but for a 'modern and dependable' NHS, a true joint venture will be required.

Nurses and health visitors working in the community and in primary care know that it is naïve to think this will just happen. Therefore, they need to understand how organisational controls can influence the way resources and efforts are combined in pursuit of mutual goals for efficient and effective healthcare. Birnbirg identifies five dimensions of interagency involvement:

Advertising 'tie-ins' ⇔ Customer supplier ⇔ Sole source supplier ⇔ Joint venture

| Low inter-organisational involvement | | High inter-organisational involvement |

Figure 7 Birnbirg's consortium of involvement.

- the degree of absolute and relative commitment
- the extent of uncertainty
- the synergy of rewards
- the degree of mutual trust
- the length of the relationship.

The relative importance of these factors varies according to the circumstances under which organisations combine, but some factors are likely to be critical in shaping controlling mechanisms. However, for a true joint venture to be established over time, mutual trust must exist as the principal controlling mechanism. In the NHS, control mechanisms covering commitment, uncertainty and symmetry of rewards are being shaped by new national policies which are summarised in Figure 8.

These mechanisms are required because the service is moving from a predominantly customer–supplier relationship to one based more on trust and partnership. The need to establish absolute and relative commitment to interagency relationships within PGC/Ts is high, but absolute and relative commitment are affected when:

- perceptions of key members are that they have more to lose than other parties, resulting in the need to seek out safeguards as protection against loss
- incentive systems do not promote behaviours that enable goals to be realised.

In the NHS the traditional contractor status of GPs has been threatened and GPs have therefore sought safeguards within the overall working agreement, resulting in controlling majorities on PCGs. Nurses and health visitors should similarly ensure that incentives are applied more widely and that they too will be recipients of incentives based on service and role development, e.g. as nurse commissioners and nurse consultants.

There is a danger that if we fail to establish trust as the principal control in a joint venture relationship, national policies will

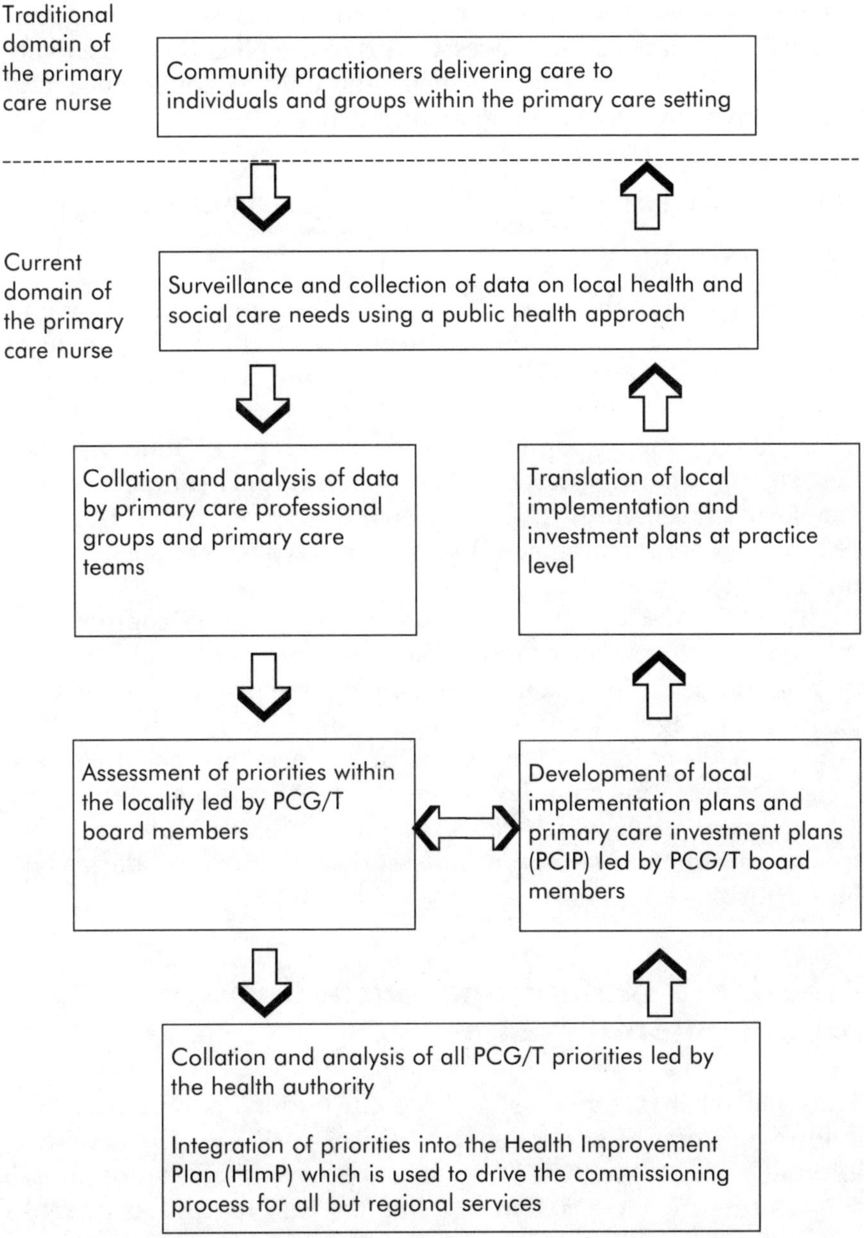

Traditional
domain of
the primary
care nurse

Community practitioners delivering care to
individuals and groups within the primary care setting

Current
domain of
the primary
care nurse

Surveillance and collection of data on local health and
social care needs using a public health approach

Collation and analysis of data
by primary care professional
groups and primary care
teams

Translation of local
implementation and
investment plans at practice
level

Assessment of priorities within
the locality led by PCG/T
board members

Development of local
implementation plans and
primary care investment plans
(PCIP) led by PCG/T board
members

Collation and analysis of all PCG/T priorities led by
the health authority

Integration of priorities into the Health Improvement
Plan (HImP) which is used to drive the commissioning
process for all but regional services

Figure 8 The process by which primary care professionals within the PCG/PCT
are expected to contribute to the formation of a local health strategy.

become new central controls. Trust needs to be based upon developing robust integrating processes and in the NHS these are likely to be associated with good financial and clinical governance, and good human resource management practices.

The need for good information technology and systems

Outside the NHS the value of using information technology and information systems (IT/IS) has been seen in the development of good inter-entity relationships. Birnbirg states that IT can facilitate relationships by building trust based upon open access to shared information. In more sophisticated relationships, IS build on existing trust by sharing knowledge that individuals can access, and enable advancement or changes in working practices. In this way IS can promote learning activities which can support the development of a learning culture.

The NHS IM&T strategy contains both IT and IS components. As part of the market economy, technology was largely used to manage information focused on measuring inputs to monitor performance against contracts. In the new NHS, outcomes and outputs will become the measures of performance and these are considerably more complex to measure. As a consequence, the development of IS which can be used to identify outcomes that transcend professional, community and acute care boundaries will be a priority.

Creating a unified approach: through organisational design

Thus far we have discussed the contribution of organisational culture and organisational control processes in creating a unified approach within the PCG/T. In addition, we stated that organisational structure had a role in enabling the PCT to fulfil its purpose or functions as one organisation.

Summarising the issues for the future

In a system where experts use the patient as a focal point, there need to be structures and processes which organise and support both individual experts and expert teams. Organisations therefore should be designed appropriately, with strong expert leadership at all levels.

Leadership should exist at both inter- and intra-professional levels and the expert system must be based on a robust set of information flows which can promote learning activities and support a learning culture. Only then can we ensure sustained continuous improvement in the development and delivery of efficient and effective healthcare.

There is debate as to whether the independent contractor status of GPs has a place in the 'New NHS'. In the future we may see an increase in the numbers of salaried GPs employed by community or PCTs. The full impact of this possible shift needs to be assessed, especially in the light of nurse prescribers and consultant nurses and the NHS Direct scheme.

Nurses and health visitors at all levels within the community services and in primary care have much to contribute to the development of a unified approach within the PCG/T, providing they develop as individuals to meet the new agenda. Only time will tell, but if the past is anything to go by, nurses and health visitors have proved themselves to be both adaptable and fast-learning. The success of PCGs and eventually PCTs will depend in large part on the development and contribution of these specialists.

References

1 Royal College of Nursing (1998) *The New Primary Care Groups: the knowledge and skills nurses need to make them a real success.* Royal College of Nursing, London.
2 Hampden-Turner C (1992) *Creating Corporate Culture: from discord to harmony.* Addison-Wesley, Reading.
3 Birnbirg J (1998) Control in inter-firm cooperative relationships. *Journal of Management Studies.* **35**(4): 421–8.

Index